JAMES WONG
HOW TO EAT BETTER

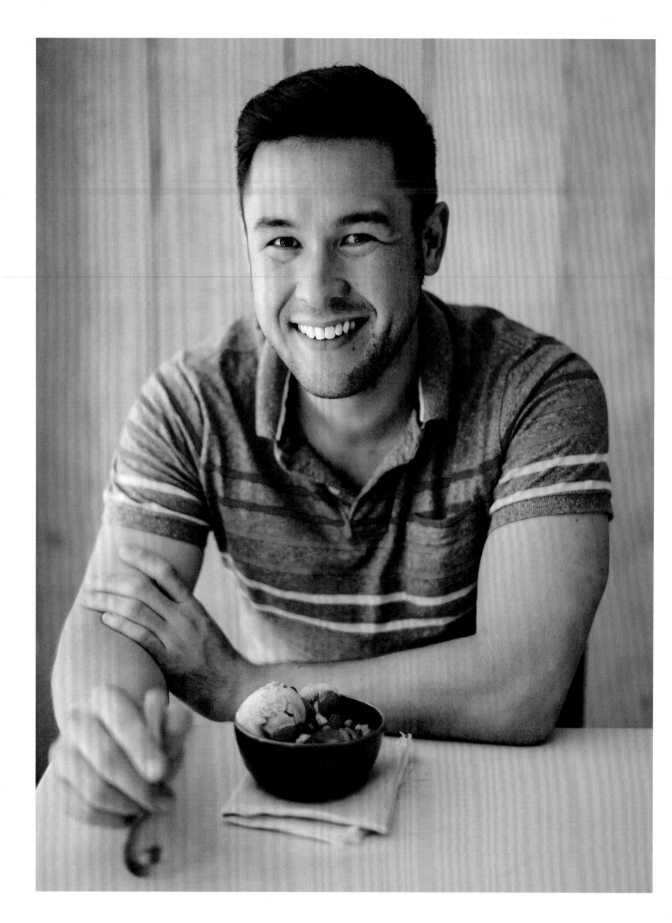

JAMES WONG
HOW TO EAT BETTER

How to Shop, Store & Cook
to Make *Any* Food a 'Superfood'

Nutritional Consultant: Dr Emma Derbyshire

MITCHELL BEAZLEY

To my wonderful friends and family for putting up with me talking
incessantly about fruit and veg for years on end. And of course to my
lovely team behind the scenes who made this book happen.

An Hachette UK Company
www.hachette.co.uk

First published in Great Britain in 2017 by
Mitchell Beazley, a division of
Octopus Publishing Group Ltd
Carmelite House
50 Victoria Embankment
London EC4Y 0DZ
www.octopusbooks.co.uk

ISBN: 978-1-78472-191-6

A CIP record for this book is available from the
British Library.

Printed and bound in Italy.

10 9 8 7 6 5 4 3 2 1

Publisher: Alison Starling
Art Director: Yasia Williams-Leedham
Senior Editor: Leanne Bryan
Project Editor: Clare Churly
Designer: Geoff Fennell
Copy-editor: Jo Murray
Senior Production Manager: Katherine Hockley

Nutritional Consultant: Dr Emma Derbyshire
Photographer: Jason Ingram
Recipe Development & Food Stylist:
   Natalie Thomson
Illustrator: Abi Read

With thanks to the following companies
for lending props for the photo shoot: Fiskars
(www.fiskars.co.uk), Iittalla (www.iittala.com),
and LSA International (www.lsa-international.com)
for the SERVE Tall Bowl.

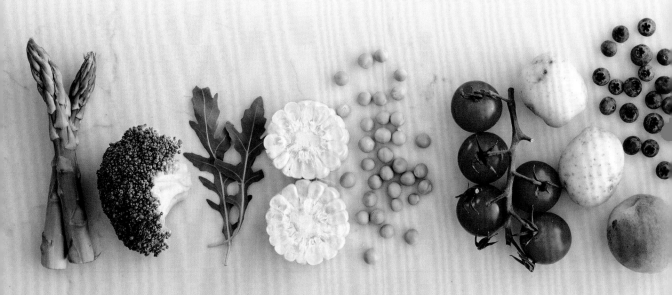

CONTENTS

Introduction 6

HOW TO MAKE ANY FOOD A 'SUPERFOOD' 8

Supercharging Nutrition 10
But What Do Scientists Know? 12
'Good' vs 'Bad' Food 14
Decoding Geek Speak 18

NOW, THE FOOD! 20

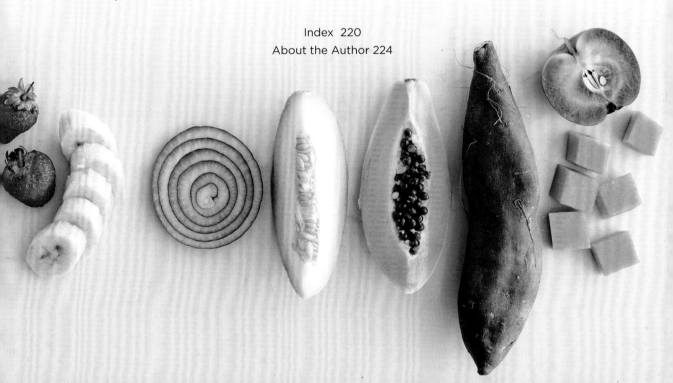

INTRODUCTION

Eating can be a confusing business. We might do it three times a day, every day, yet somehow knowing how to eat healthily suddenly seems to have become enormously complicated. Take one look at a 'wellness' blog or step into a health-food store, for example, and you'll learn that it's *essential* that all sorts of everyday foods are immediately banned from our diets – wheat, dairy, potatoes – in fact, it seems, anything that's a common, affordable staple, really. In their place we apparently need to seek out fancy 'superfood' ingredients from the depths of the Amazon or the high Himalayas. Of course, these will also need to be organic and preferably have the words 'heritage' or 'artisan' on the packet. After all, being exclusive and expensive must mean a food is better for you, right?

However, there is a simpler way, and one that's actually based on solid science. And the best news is, you already know it: as dieticians and doctors have been telling us for years, eat lots of fruit, veg and whole grains, and go easy on the red meat, fat and sugar. Admittedly, it doesn't make for dramatic headlines or scandalous-sounding narratives, but this advice really hasn't changed and neither have the decades of rigorous research upon which it's based. Phew!

But what if a little kitchen science could dramatically boost the nutrition in the healthy, everyday ingredients you love simply by how you choose to SELECT, STORE and COOK them? We are talking measurably more vitamins, minerals, fibre, antioxidants and a whole host of other benefits in everything from apples and oranges to pasta and coffee. In fact, there are whole academic libraries full of scientific studies from around the world that have looked into how to do just that for every ingredient going. As a plant scientist with a lifelong food fixation, I love a challenge, so I have spent the last two years trawling through nearly 3,000 such papers, translating the dense academic geek speak into practical tips and tricks to send the nutrition in pretty much any plant-based ingredient soaring.

Pop your punnet of mushrooms on a sunny windowsill for an hour or two and get 100 times more vitamin D2. Simmer up blueberries into a tasty 3-minute compote and get 100 per cent more antioxidants than scoffing them raw. Pick pink grapefruit over white and you get fruit that not only tastes sweeter, but also has 34 times the vitamin A, plus a generous dose of antioxidant lycopene to boot. No fads, no obscure ingredients, no damn spiralizer, just ordinary, everyday food made better. This book is not about what to eat, but how to eat the foods you love to get the very most out of them – all backed by the very best scientific evidence going.

Ladies and gents, here's how to make almost any food a 'superfood'...

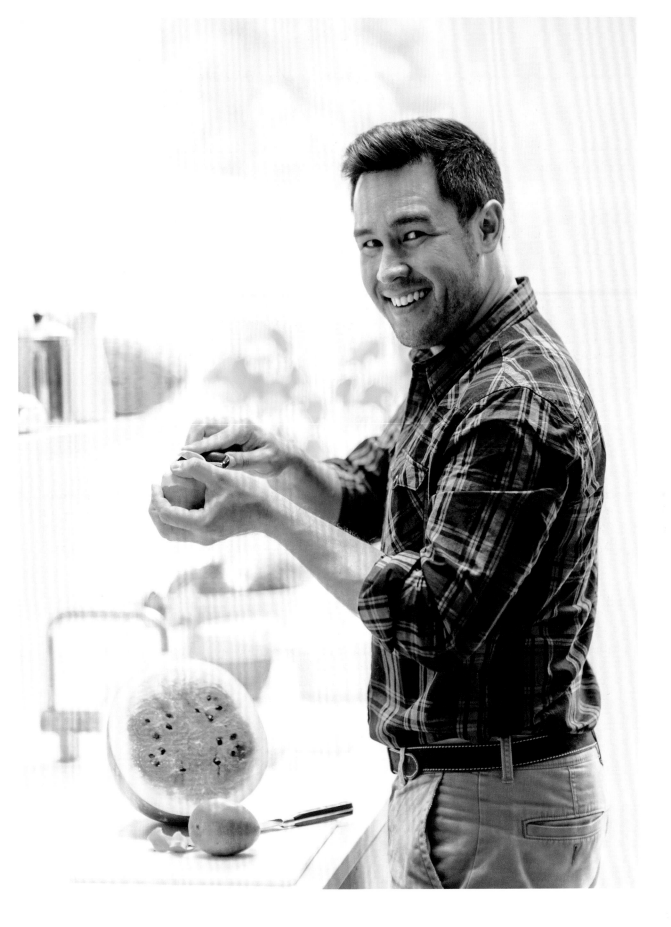

HOW TO MAKE ANY FOOD A 'SUPERFOOD'

SUPERCHARGING NUTRITION

Improving the nutritional benefits of crops really isn't rocket science, it's just about how you choose to SELECT, STORE and COOK them. Little changes can have surprising impacts. I know this might sound a little too good to be true, so here is the low-down on how it works.

SELECT

We tend to think of ingredients as generic objects whose nutritional value is fixed and constant. I mean, an apple is an apple, is an apple. Simple, right? But what if I were to tell you that some varieties can contain several times the antioxidant levels of others sitting on the very same shelf? Pick a Red Delicious over an Empire, for example, and get two and a half times the potential antioxidant benefit for zero extra work or cost. The same thing applies to pretty much every plant-based ingredient, from spuds and grapes to rice and even instant coffee. You see, not all crops were created equal. With a plant's unique genetics being the single biggest determining factor behind their internal chemistry and therefore nutritional value, knowing how to select them can make a phenomenal difference.

STORE

For me, the fascinating thing about fruit and veg is that even once harvested they are still alive and carry on responding to their surrounding environment with ever-changing internal chemistry – just like all living plants. Store your apples on a sunny kitchen windowsill instead of in the light-less fridge, for example, and the skin of the fruit can react to the UV rays by kicking out loads more protective polyphenols plus six times the vitamin C. Tomatoes can detect that they have been detached from the plant and will respond by becoming redder, more fragrant and higher in an important antioxidant called lycopene, but only if kept at above 10°C. Any lower and these reactions just won't happen, so store them on the work surface.

On the other hand, broccoli can lose an astonishing 80 per cent of its cancer-fighting chemicals in the few days it takes to hit the shelf, so it's worth scoffing this as soon as you get it home. If you buy it wrapped in plastic and keep it well chilled, however, this decline is halted dead in its tracks and the broccoli retains almost all of its original antioxidant content. Understanding how to store your fruit and veg can genuinely give you way more nutrition for really no additional effort.

COOK

There seems to be an increasingly popular idea that eating fruit and veg raw is the healthiest possible option. Sounds intuitively plausible, doesn't it? Yet take a crisp, leafy spinach salad and whack it in a pan for a few minutes and its vitamin A levels shoot up three times (and that's before we even mention that because spinach wilts down so much on cooking, one serving of cooked greens can contain up to five servings of raw). The exact same phenomenon of cooking increasing a food's nutritional content also occurs in carrots, winter squashes, tomatoes and sweet potatoes too.

However, this same blast of heat can slash the benefits of other crops, such as garlic, onions and broccoli, making them measurably more nutrient dense when raw. Does the prospect of crunching on raw broccoli fill you with dread? No problem, adding a tiny bit of mustard triggers a natural chemical reaction that – as if by magic – makes the cooked stuff just as good as fresh, while simultaneously boosting its flavour (see page 40). Fancy a knob of butter on that sweet potato? Go ahead. It makes its vitamin A even more absorbable. So you can see, knowing how to cook fruit and veg, and what tasty stuff to serve them with, can not only retain their benefits but even substantially improve them.

MY PROMISE

For almost every crop going, this book will show you how these three factors, SELECT, STORE and COOK, can work together to give nutrition a major boost. These aren't hard and fast rules that you need to stick to like gospel, though, just tips and tricks based on the best available scientific evidence. You can pick and choose which ones work best for your taste, time availability and lifestyle. It doesn't matter, for example, if you don't like cherry tomatoes (which have more healthy lycopene than beefsteaks); whichever variety you pick, tomatoes will still have more lycopene if you choose to cook them. This book is all about practical, real-world advice that can work for anyone. Frankly, all fruit, veg and whole grains are good for you; I have provided a bunch of simple ideas on how you can make them even better.

AT-A-GLANCE SYMBOLS

These symbols will help you to quickly navigate the book to find the key information about the nutritional benefits of each crop and the best ways to select, store and cook the ingredient.

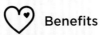 Benefits Store

 Select Cook

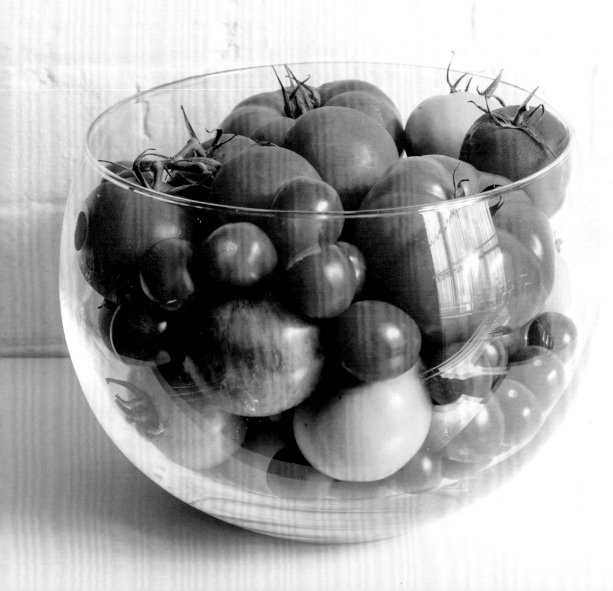

BUT WHAT DO SCIENTISTS KNOW?

My mum is weary of nutritional advice and, after reading recent newspaper reports, has ended up asking: 'If these blinking scientists know everything, how come they keep changing their minds?' And even as a scientist myself, I can see her point. If one month a headline definitively proclaims that 'eating bacon poses as great a cancer risk as smoking' and a few months later another describes bacon as being 'full of healthy fats' and 'great for weight loss' (complete with bacon-heavy recipes), it is easy to understand why people can be left confused and frustrated – especially if the two opposing stories both claim to be backed by the latest scientific evidence and are even published in the same paper! So what's going on here?

The funny thing is that, despite the headlines, overall dietary advice hasn't changed very much in decades and, as I mentioned earlier, this is primarily because the weight of objective, rigorous evidence that underpins it hasn't changed either. You see, scientists don't really change their minds that often, journalists however are quite a different story – they are called *news*papers, after all. Unfortunately, 'researchers say the same things they have said all along' is hardly enticing clickbait, and with thousands of studies to pick from around the world, it is very easy for the press to selectively pick and choose the ones with findings that appear to fit a much more exciting, surprising or otherwise novel narrative – even if it isn't really very accurate. Frequently the very early results from pilot studies can make headlines, proclaimed as incontrovertible 'shocking truths', even if the very authors of the studies have gone to great lengths to highlight their limitations. Perhaps most important of all, and something not all non-scientists will know, is that not all studies carry equal weight – some types simply provide much stronger evidence than others.

As I believe readers deserve more than to just take my word for it, I have cited a broad range of studies throughout this book. Understanding what the different types of research are and the strength of the evidence they provide will hopefully give you an insight into how researchers arrive at their conclusions, and will help you sift through fact and fantasy in the next nutrition headline. Here's why some evidence is better than others.

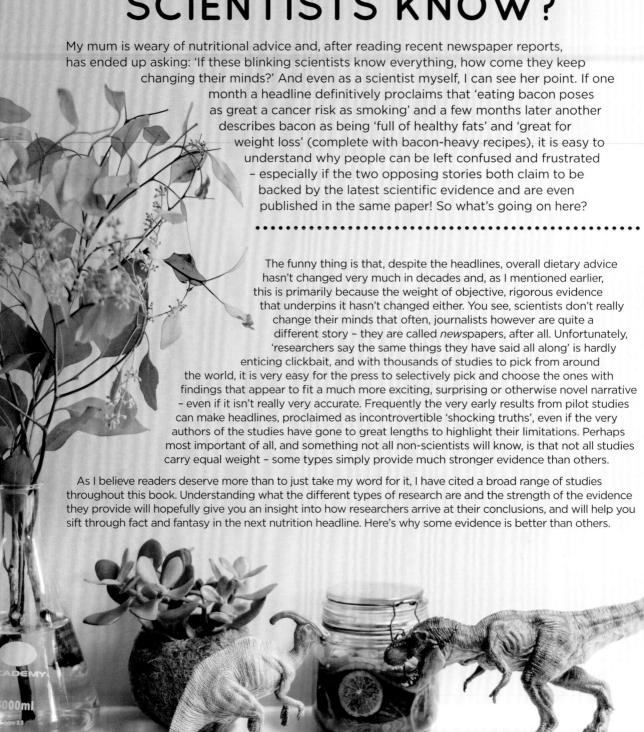

THE HIERARCHY OF NUTRITIONAL EVIDENCE

TYPE OF STUDY

WHAT THIS MEANS

Systematic reviews are studies of studies that pool together the results of loads of the best-quality trials and examine them to see if they can find a consistent pattern.

A clear, unbiased overview of the best available info we have so far, reviewing loads of studies helps detect and eliminate any red herrings. As the hallmark of good science is reproducability, these reviews are about as rigorous as it gets.

Clinical trials serve people a regular dose of a specific food/compound in a carefully controlled setting and see if it affects their health. Some trials are far more carefully controlled than others, meaning their results are more reliable.

The more people in a study, the more reliable its findings are likely to be, too, which helps iron out any fluke results. For this reason, it is important to look at not only a clinical study's findings, but also its methods. In this book, I have done this for you. If a study has intriguing results but only tested a tiny number of people, I'll make it clear.

Observational studies carefully track the habits of a large population of people to see if there are associations between eating certain foods and certain health outcomes.

The Achilles heel of these studies is that they can only show associations, not actually prove cause and effect. For example, sales of sun cream and ice cream both rise in the summer, but one does not cause the other. As the geeks say, 'correlation does not equal causation'.

Animal studies give lab animals a regular dose of a food and measure the effects on their health.

These studies can be a really useful tool to identify promising leads, but they have a simple flaw: humans aren't lab rats. This means the results often aren't replicable when you run the same experiment in people. In fact, as few as 30 per cent of the findings of animal and test-tube studies are later reflected in human subjects. They can still point out useful clues – if taken with a pinch of salt.

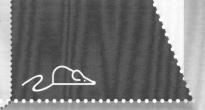

Test-tube studies apply extracts of a food to isolated cells or chemical models of parts of the human body and see what the results are.

We are even further removed from blobs of cultured cells in a petri dish than we are from lab rats, of course. As one of my dietician heroes says, 'What happens in the test tube stays in the test tube.' Useful as a first step to find initial tip-offs, but far, far away from conclusive evidence. Take with an even larger pinch of salt.

QUALITY OF EVIDENCE

'GOOD' VS 'BAD' FOOD

I wrote this section sitting on a train. In front of me were a group of smart, 20-something women, lunch boxes on their knees, all talking about food. Now, I am not some kind of weirdo who makes a habit of transcribing strangers' conversations but, in the space of ten minutes, I made a note of some of the words they used to describe what they were eating: 'clean', 'junk', 'virtuous', 'naughty', 'good', 'bad', 'pure' and 'guilt'. As a scientist, I find these word choices fascinating. To me they sound far more like ethical, almost religious, proclamations than simple sandwich choices. Yet these women are by no means unique. If you listen carefully, pretty much any discussion about food is crammed with emotionally charged words, and when we start talking nutrition, adjectives can suddenly become morally loaded. It's almost as if what we pick for dinner somehow makes us better (or worse) people.

One curious side effect of attaching moral labels to food is that it can cause us to damage our health, paradoxically often in the pursuit of well-being. It can make us avoid 'bad' foods that can make valuable additions to our diet, limiting our intake of key nutrients, while conversely causing us to believe 'good' foods are healthier than they actually are. In this section, I outline what I feel are the four biggest nutritional myths of 'good' and 'bad' foods today.

PROCESSED FOODS ARE 'BAD'

This one seems a no-brainer, right? Fresh, home-cooked meals have got to be better than processed 'junk'. Many writers – including several doctors I know – claim the single most important thing you can do for your health is to cook at home and avoid all processed foods. There are even catchy mantras like: 'Processed foods were invented by #BigFood to make them wealthy. Nature invented whole #realfood to make us healthy!'

But here's the inconvenient truth. Cooking is a process. As is chewing. In fact, far from being a modern spectre conspiring to damage human health, food processing is as old as our species – representing the earliest human technology. But can you really compare the kind of cooking that goes on in my kitchen with what happens in giant industrial assembly lines? Well, yes, you can. The supermarket ready-meal ravioli I had for lunch contains only wheat flour, eggs, water, cheese, spinach, salt and spices, and is made using the same processes that I would use at home, albeit significantly scaled up. Chemically, and therefore nutritionally, there is essentially no meaningful difference. Whether made in a kitchen or in a factory, what matters to our bodies is what it contains, not where it was made.

This reality was made strikingly clear in a study published in *The British Medical Journal*, which compared 100 recipes from bestselling cookbooks by top TV chefs (including those whose home cooking is sometimes perceived as the healthy choice) with 100 supermarket ready meals. The processed foods contained far less sugar, calories and fat (including a quarter less saturated fat) than the home-cooked recipes and as much as twice the fibre. This does somewhat question the idea that simply the location of a food's production makes a difference to its nutritional outcomes.

In fact, many heavily processed foods are actually measurably more nutritious than less processed alternatives. The pressure-steaming method used to create parboiled rice, for example, causes it to retain higher levels of B vitamins, niacin, riboflavin and thiamine. Golden raisins treated with the (100 per cent safe) preservative sulphur dioxide to retain their original colour, also retain three times the antioxidants as a direct consequence. Even the ready-made fruit salad I once read as being 'soaked in acid', in a tabloid's 'shocking truth' exposé, is significantly higher in vitamin C than homemade. Why? Well the 'acid' in question is ascorbic acid, the chemical name for vitamin C. A more truthful headline would have read 'Shop-bought fruit salad comes with added vitamin C'. But I guess that just doesn't sound as scary.

To me, this highlights one of the dangers of illogically demonizing processed foods: it can heavily skew our perception of a food's nutritional value. Compared to the shop-bought alternative, cake is not any healthier if it's homemade using 'real ingredients'. It is still cake and your body will treat it just the same. Likewise, sweets, sugary cereals, crisps and ice cream aren't great choices to base your diet on, not because they are processed 'fake foods', but because of the chemical constituents they are made up of.

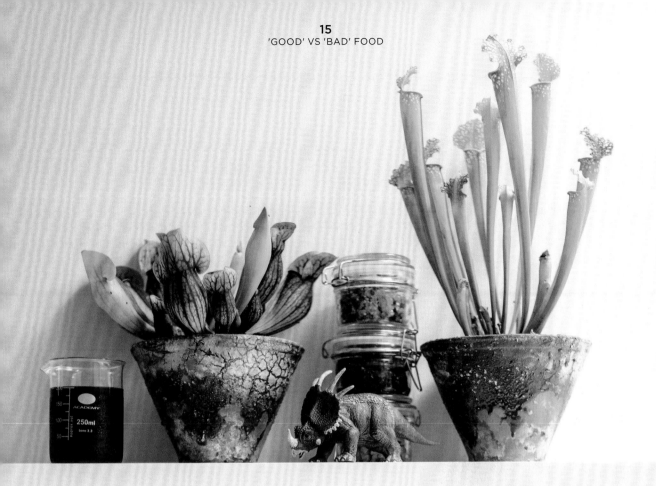

One of the curious things about the demonization of processed foods is that people who are against them tend to apply this label quite inconsistently and only to things they happen to ideologically disapprove of. My local health-food store, for example, has a huge sign that reads 'Say NO to processed foods and added sugars'. Below it, the 'paleo granola' – a sort of grain-free breakfast 'cereal' – that can contain per 100g up to twice the sugar of fizzy cola and more fat than a pork pie. It is, of course, also a processed food. According to scientific definitions used by government health agencies, processed foods make up the vast majority of the supermarket's shelf space.

ORGANIC IS 'GOOD'

'Did you know? Switching to organic is the same as adding 2 portions to your 5-A-Day?' proudly boasts the flyer for an organic box scheme. Assertions like this are so commonly repeated about organic food that it seems they must be true. But what evidence are they based on?

I decided to put this to the company. In its reply, it said the claim was based on a study from Newcastle University that found that organically grown fruit and veg contained up to twice the levels of antioxidants as conventionally grown. And sure enough, this paper does exist. It crunched the numbers of hundreds of previous studies comparing organic and conventional produce. The study found that, when viewed as a whole, there was little difference in the vitamin and mineral content between organic and conventional crops (this information was not included in the flyer). While some vitamins could be higher in organic, other vitamins and minerals were much lower. That doesn't sound like switching to organic is the same as adding two portions to your 5-a-day to me!

Now admittedly, the study also reported that the organically grown fruit and veg had up to 60 per cent more antioxidants. However, its results are at odds with three other similar reviews that consistently found little or no meaningful difference between the two growing methods in fruit and veg. Remember, the hallmark of good science is its reproducibility. In fact, the study has been widely criticized by academics for poor methodology and overstating the public health significance of this difference. For example, the research went to great lengths to investigate residues of synthetic pesticides used in conventional agriculture, but chose not to look at potentially equally toxic pesticides of natural origin used by organic farmers. While the results in the main body of the paper also found organic crops to be lower in fibre, protein and potentially heart-healthy dietary nitrates, these findings were not highlighted to anywhere near the same extent as organic's apparent antioxidant benefits. The study's independence has also been queried as it was partially funded by a charity whose mission statement is to promote organic agriculture. But, of course, this could be just a coincidence.

On balance, while some studies do suggest that organic crops can be higher in certain nutrients, others show the exact opposite, creating a body of evidence that is highly contradictory. It is simply impossible to claim organic fruit and vegetables are more nutrient dense overall without picking and choosing studies to prove your point while conspicuously ignoring others. What we do know about organic crops for certain is that they tend to be more expensive, sometimes significantly more so. Forking out a little more for organic crops is unlikely to do any harm, but despite the marketeers' best efforts, it won't mean you can get away with just eating less fruit and veg to get your 5-a-day.

LOCAL & IN SEASON ARE 'GOOD'

It's rare that a nutrition-based headline really surprises me, but when I read that traditional British fruits are far healthier than modern imported ones,

I was fascinated to find out why. According to this press story, imported fruit like oranges and bananas – apparently a rarity 50 years ago – are far too high in sugar compared to traditional tart British fruit like gooseberries and apples. Even in the case of good old English apples, we now prefer modern imported varieties that are apparently packed with far more of the sweet stuff than old British favourites, and this all comes at an adverse cost to our health. Articles asserting this 'local is better' mantra are not unusual, and are usually tied in with the gospel of 'traditional is better'. So let's take a closer look at this claim.

Well, it turns out all four fruits mentioned in the press article actually contain very similar amounts of the sweet stuff – as do most fruit – hovering around 10 per cent. Even intensely tart British apples like Bramley have comparatively similar levels of sugar to sweeter-tasting imported apples, it's just that they also have as much as twice the acid, which masks the taste of the sugar. Their intense sourness does however mean it's often also necessary to add sugar to them to make them palatable, which is probably why the article (on the evils of over-sugary imported fruit) ended in a crumble recipe! (Brilliant.) With regards to the past, I should perhaps point out that oranges and bananas were common foodstuffs in 1960s Britain. With a longer season and cheaper price than gooseberries, for example, they have been more frequently consumed since as early as the turn of the century.

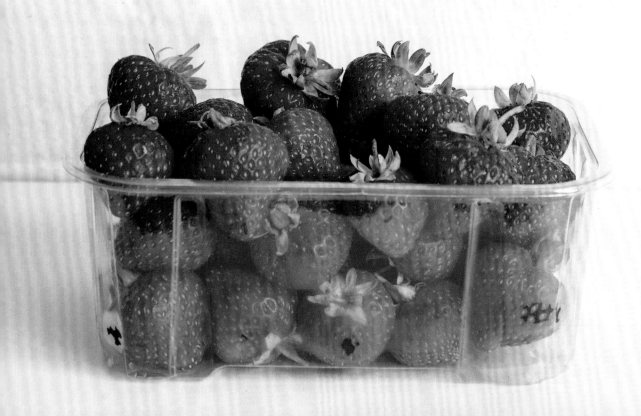

Of course, certain crops can be far more nutritious depending on local conditions. For example, tomatoes grown in the sun-soaked Mediterranean have been shown to have higher levels of the antioxidant lycopene than ones grown in cooler climates. This means, for Italians, local tomatoes may indeed be healthier, but for people living in, say, Sweden not so much. The idea that the proximity of a food's origin to the person consuming it is a direct indicator of nutritional content is really not based on any sound logic. Indeed, even from an environmental standpoint, because as little as 6 per cent of a food's carbon footprint is generated by transport, German-grown tomatoes reared in heated, lit greenhouses on the shelves of local supermarkets are likely to have burned just as much if not more fossil fuel than those trucked up from sunny Spain.

Last but not least there is also an inherent problem with defining 'local'. For many people this means the same country. Yet for me as a Londoner, imported Belgian tomatoes actually are more 'local' in a geographical sense than British tomatoes grown in Cornwall. In short, if you want to support growers situated within your own country that's great; however, if you think shopping 'local' will automatically mean healthier, tastier or more eco-friendly food, this is not always the case and, frequently, it is the exact opposite.

Wind back time 50 or 100 years ago and, apart from eating more locally, we also tended to eat more seasonally. The popular argument here is that as an obvious consequence of both, we would have been healthier. Yet 100 years ago, far from being a golden age of public health, hunger and malnutrition were rife. The limited availability of foods in the winter months, and particularly the lack of diversity, made nutrient deficiencies commonplace. In the 1950s in rural Wales, my grandparents ate only the veg they could grow, so their options at breakfast, lunch and dinner were limited to just six crops for nearly half the year – cabbage, swedes, carrots, turnips, spuds and parsnips – which was not only culinarily boring (as my mum frequently attests), but also nutritionally far more limited. For this reason, since the dawn of time humans have been trying to find ways to grow, store and preserve foods to extend their season far beyond their natural range. In fact, the miracle of modern technology means we have never had access to a greater variety of safe, nutritious and affordable food. Even when you compare like-for-like examples of, say, blueberries imported in winter from Chile versus ones harvested in season on your doorstep, they still contain essentially all the same vitamins and minerals. In short? Eating seasonally is fine if you want to, but it isn't necessarily any healthier.

CARBS ARE 'BAD'

It might have been fat in the 1980s, but today it seems carbs are now well and truly our foodie villain *du jour*. Frequently attributed to be the central cause of some of the worst health afflictions to plague the modern world, carbs are getting the blame for everything from soaring obesity rates to diabetes in books and blogs everywhere. Many of these commentators are also deeply critical of conventional evidence-based diet advice, questioning why all of society doesn't switch to a low-carb regime.

There is a thorn in the side of this argument however, and that is that diets based on complex carbohydrates pre-date the modern rise of these diet-related diseases by tens of thousands of years. In fact, with the rise of protein and fat in industrialized diets the total portion of carbs in many diets has actually fallen in recent years, making it kind of hard to pin the blame for this on them. You see, consuming more calories than your body uses in our increasingly sedentary lives is the ultimate cause of weight gain, and this can come from any food group, not just carbs.

But before we even get into the risks of missing out on essential nutrients, such as fibre, there is a much more simple reason why society can't abandon carbs. All complex human civilizations independently evolved eating carbohydrate-rich foods – in particular grains – as their key energy source because these crops yield maximum calories per minimum land area. It's about simple maths. Base your calorie intake on beef instead of rice, wheat or potatoes and you need roughly 100 times more land. Sadly, we just don't have an extra planet.

What about people with diabetes? Well according to a major review by respected health-charity Diabetes UK there is indeed good evidence that going low carb can improve the health of diabetics in the short term. But this is simply because low-carb diets reduce the total calories people tend to consume, resulting in short-term weight loss. Losing weight by any means (low carb or not) has been shown to improve the health of diabetics too. In the long term however the researchers found a lack of evidence for the benefit (and safety) of low-carb diets.

Current scientific consensus, based on the vast weight of evidence from thousands of studies from around the world, recommends that carbs make up half of our total calorie intake, more than any other food group. This book will show you the most nutrient-dense types and how best to prepare them.

DECODING GEEK SPEAK

I have tried to avoid the temptation to lapse into dense academic geek speak in this book, but I am also a firm believer that using correct terminology can be really helpful to give newbies a clear understanding of how the science behind these tips and tricks actually works. To help you out, here's a quick run-down of the technical terms you might come across in the following pages. Hopefully you won't need it, as I have tried to weave explanations into the text, but it may be a handy reference to flick back to if you need clarification.

WHAT ARE NUTRIENTS?

Nutrients are substances that provide nourishment essential for growth and the maintenance of life. There are three broad classes of these: vitamins, minerals and phytonutrients. While there have been decades of research and well-established dietary guidelines for the exact amounts of vitamins and minerals we need, other compounds in plants known as phytonutrients have only become of interest to researchers more recently and are often overlooked. Here's how the three break down:

Vitamins

Vitamins are chemicals made by plants and animals that human bodies need to function, yet sadly we can't produce all of the vitamins that we need. To stay healthy we need to essentially steal them from other species by consuming these through our diets.

Minerals

Minerals exist in rocks and soil, and are sucked up by plants through their roots. From there they enter the food chain either directly, when we consume plants, or indirectly from animals that have eaten these plants. We need both to get both vitamins and minerals through our diets in the correct amounts in order to survive. Without them our bodies would soon cease to function.

Phytonutrients

Phytonutrients are chemicals produced by plants that have beneficial effects on health when we eat them. Unlike vitamins however, they are not absolutely necessary for our immediate survival. You can go for months or even years without eating some of these phytonutrients and still stay alive, but diets rich in these chemicals are associated with preventing many degenerative diseases and promoting better overall health.

There are loads of different types of phytonutrients, from polyphenols to carotenes that have wide-ranging biological effects we are still only beginning to understand, which means they have attracted a huge degree of scientific interest in recent years. Many of the chemicals I focus on in this book, following the available science, belong to this group.

- **Polyphenols** are a group of closely related chemicals usually produced by plants to help protect themselves. Plants can't run away or hide from external threats, so they have developed chemical defences as an entirely different evolutionary strategy. These compounds can do stuff like shield their delicate cells from harmful ultra-violet rays, as in the case of bright purple and red pigments like anthocyanins, that are believed to give blueberries their health benefits. Many other polyphenols are responsible for the flavour and scent of plants, designed to either deter pests or attract animals that can help pollinate their flowers or spread their seeds. Others are antibacterial or antifungal agents designed to fight off disease. Some are signalling chemicals that control the complex chemical reactions that go on in plants, like quercetin which is believed to give onions, citrus and apples part of their associated health benefits. There are hundreds of polyphenols out there!

- **Carotenes** are bright yellow and orange pigments that serve loads of different functions in plants, from shielding fruit from UV damage (just like the anthocyanins mentioned above), to bouncing light on to exactly the part of the leaves where it is needed for photosynthesis to take place. There are lots of different types, many of which are believed to have health benefits such as protecting eye health, potentially lowering cancer risk, having antioxidant effects, with some even convertible by the body into vitamin A. This group includes the betacarotene that gives pumpkins their colour, alpha carotenes that make carrots orange and lycopene which makes both tomatoes and watermelons red. In fact, most orange and red fruit and veg contain a mix of several different types of carotenes.

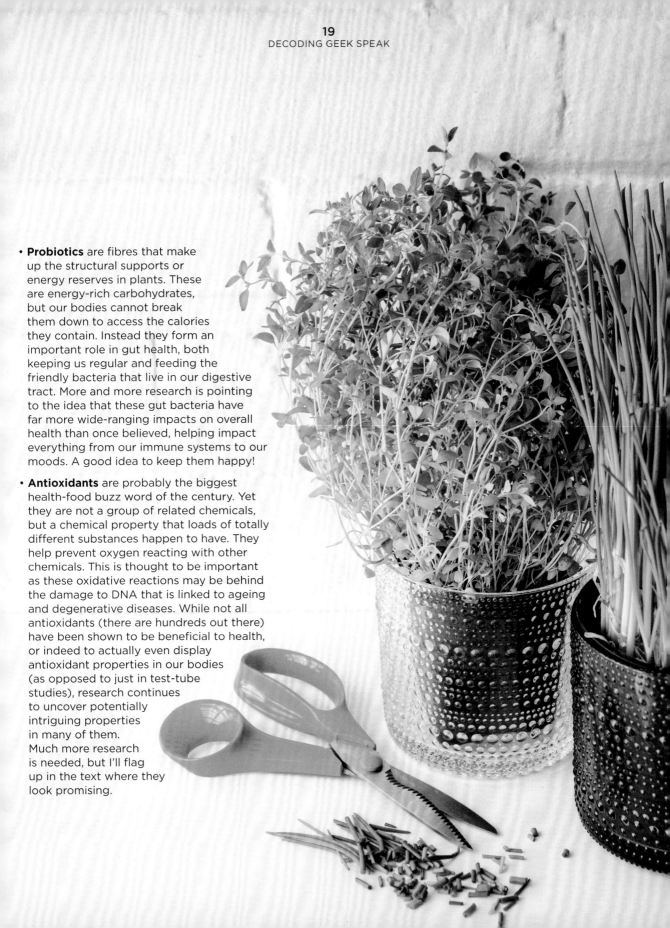

• **Probiotics** are fibres that make up the structural supports or energy reserves in plants. These are energy-rich carbohydrates, but our bodies cannot break them down to access the calories they contain. Instead they form an important role in gut health, both keeping us regular and feeding the friendly bacteria that live in our digestive tract. More and more research is pointing to the idea that these gut bacteria have far more wide-ranging impacts on overall health than once believed, helping impact everything from our immune systems to our moods. A good idea to keep them happy!

• **Antioxidants** are probably the biggest health-food buzz word of the century. Yet they are not a group of related chemicals, but a chemical property that loads of totally different substances happen to have. They help prevent oxygen reacting with other chemicals. This is thought to be important as these oxidative reactions may be behind the damage to DNA that is linked to ageing and degenerative diseases. While not all antioxidants (there are hundreds out there) have been shown to be beneficial to health, or indeed to actually even display antioxidant properties in our bodies (as opposed to just in test-tube studies), research continues to uncover potentially intriguing properties in many of them. Much more research is needed, but I'll flag up in the text where they look promising.

NOW, THE FOOD!

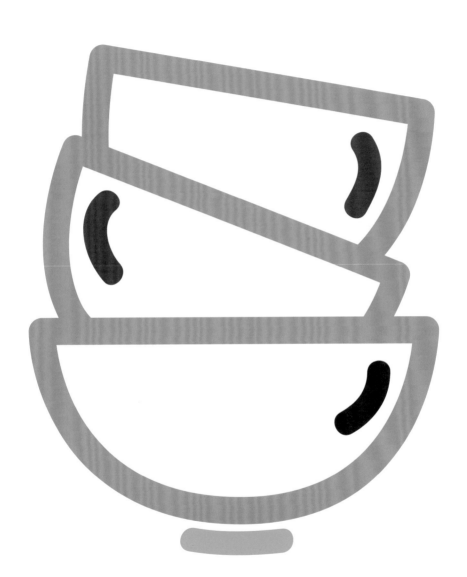

TOMATOES

Tomatoes are a great source of vitamins A and C, plus they contain a healthy dose of fibre – just like loads of other fruit and veg – but two things set them apart from the rest. First, we eat an awful lot of them. In the United States, for example, they are second only to spuds in popularity, with these two crops alone making up more than half of all vegetables consumed in the country. Secondly, tomatoes and their products are by far the richest dietary source of a phytonutrient known as lycopene, the carotene pigment responsible for their red colour, which has attracted keen interest from scientists all over the world for its potential health benefits. Combine an unrivalled source of a promising phytonutrient in a super-popular package and you could have a pretty potent mix on your hands. Here's the latest evidence on making the most of them.

♡ SKIN PROTECTION

UV damage is one of the leading causes of skin wrinkling and can lead to the development of skin cancers. Our bodies naturally produce their own antioxidant defence chemicals to help shield our skin cells from the ravages of the sun, but could consuming extra antioxidants like lycopene through our diet help further protect against this damage?

One small study at the University of Manchester aimed to find out by supplementing the diets of a group of women with either a daily dose of 55g (about 4 tablespoons) of concentrated tomato purée or a placebo. After 3 months, the tomato eaters were found to possess a surprising 33 per cent higher protection against sunburn when subjected to UV light, the equivalent of that provided by a very low-factor sunscreen. But this internal defence didn't end there; the tomato-rich diet also appeared to have reduced the damage to DNA that is linked to skin ageing. And when the researchers studied skin samples taken from the women, those from the tomato group were found to have significantly higher levels of procollagen, the protein responsible for the firmness of youthful skin, which declines as we get older. Perhaps the most surprising thing is that this amount of lycopene was hardly excessive: we are talking about the amount found in an average serving of pasta sauce, a 300ml glass of tomato juice or a bowl of tomato soup, for example, which is easily doable for most people.

♡ CANCER RISK

Several large observational studies that have tracked the diets of tens of thousands of people suggest that those with lycopene-rich diets have a significantly reduced incidence of certain types of cancer. One Harvard University study, for example, found that those with the highest intakes

35%
lower risk
of **prostate
cancer**

of tomatoes and their products had a 35 per cent lower risk of prostate cancer, including a 53 per cent lower risk of the most aggressive forms.

Reviews focusing on other cancers also found a similar association between tomato consumption and a lowered risk of developing stomach and lung cancers. While we still don't know for sure whether this risk reduction is related to lycopene itself, some other compound in tomatoes or even another as yet unknown factor associated with lycopene-rich diets, considerable scientific interest in this compound's potential protective effects continues. I for one can't wait to find out more.

♡ HEART HEALTH & STROKE

In a review of seven studies involving over 100,000 people, researchers reported that those with the highest lycopene consumption had almost a 20 per cent reduced risk of stroke. Add this to the fact that another such study at Italy's Catholic University School of Medicine noted a significant reduction in the risk of heart disease in tomato lovers, then digging into a Bolognese seems an even more attractive idea.

20%
lower risk
of **stroke**

LOCAL ISN'T ALWAYS BETTER

One of the key functions of lycopene in plants is to act as a biological sunscreen, protecting their sensitive tissues from damaging solar radiation. The more sunshine there is, the more good stuff you get.

In fact, according to University College Cork, up to three times more when you pick tomatoes grown in the sunny Med over those grown under the overcast skies of northern Europe.

LITTLE FRUIT, BIG NUTRITION

The phytonutrients in tomatoes are not distributed uniformly across the fruit, but concentrated largely in their skin. When talking lycopene, for example, there is as much as five times more in the skin than in the juicy pulp. But the story doesn't end there. A study at the University of Glasgow discovered that 98 per cent of the flavonols (anti-inflammatory compounds that can reduce cholesterol and blood pressure and may even prevent against certain types of cancer) are found in this incredibly thin coating. OK, most of us don't go to the bother of peeling tomatoes, so why is this relevant? Well, it's all about variety choice.

Cherry types

The small size of mini cherry types gives them a far greater surface area and therefore much more skin gram for gram than their big, beefsteak cousins, making them potentially far denser in these phytonutrients. In fact, the Glasgow study found that simply picking cherry tomatoes over regular round types could give you twice as many flavonols. Similar results have been found in a number of studies for the red pigment lycopene, too, with cherry types consistently having on average about twice the amount of lycopene. Compare the palest regular tomatoes with the very reddest cherry types and this difference could be more than 15 times, according to a large trial at Texas A&M University.

Cherry tomatoes are also generally sweeter and much richer flavoured than the bigger types. This is because the chemical responsible for the savoury, umami flavour of tomatoes is concentrated in the gel that surrounds their many seeds, containing six times as much as the flesh that beefsteaks proportionately have more of. Pick cherry types and get better flavour and loads more phytonutrients. Boom!

THE FRIDGE SPELLS DOOM

Even once detached from the plant, tomato fruit will continue to ripen, becoming sweeter, more aromatic, redder and, as a consequence, much higher in lycopene. In fact, tomatoes can almost double their lycopene levels if stored at room temperature for a week or two according to a Japanese–Indonesian research team.

However, the chemical reactions responsible for this transformation will not occur below 10°C. Tomatoes are, after all, a subtropical fruit. So please, always store them on the work surface.

2x
the **lycopene**
if stored on the
counter

Baby plum types

Want even more? Baby plum tomatoes could well kick the lycopene levels up yet another notch, and again it's all about surface area. Shrink a spherical fruit and its ratio of skin to flesh increases; stretch it to an egg shape and the ratio increases further still. It should be no surprise then that egg-shaped baby plums can have 30 per cent more lycopene than spherical cherry tomatoes, not to mention less acid and a deeper red colour, according to researchers at Italy's University of Catania. The same principle appears to be even more pronounced in regular plum tomatoes, which on average have higher levels than similarly sized round tomatoes, with some plums having up to three times more lycopene gram for gram, according to the United States Department of Agriculture (USDA).

FEWER PHYTONUTRIENTS ➤ **MORE PHYTONUTRIENTS** ➤

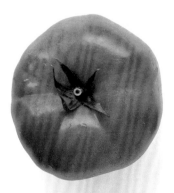

Beefsteak tomatoes

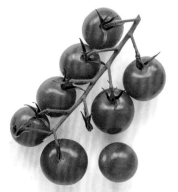

Cherry tomatoes

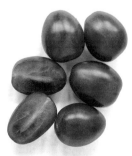

Baby plum tomatoes

GIVE GREEN A GO

Unripe tomatoes and varieties that maintain their emerald hue even when ripe contain little or no lycopene, but they are packed full of two other compounds – tomatine and tomatidine (evidently, scientists aren't hugely creative when it comes to naming new chemicals!) – which some emerging studies suggest may have intriguing benefits. Research at the University of Iowa found that in mice, tomatidine not only was capable of reducing muscle wasting (a common and debilitating condition in humans) but could even reverse it. The critters given tomatidine actually saw an increase in muscle mass, strength and exercise capacity, with similar results also being observed in human muscle cells cultivated in test tubes.

One study published in the *Journal of Agricultural and Food Chemistry* found that tomatine was highly effective in inhibiting the growth of breast, colon, gastric and liver cancer cells, in test tubes at least, leading the researchers to conclude that 'consumers may benefit by eating not only high-lycopene red tomatoes but also green'.

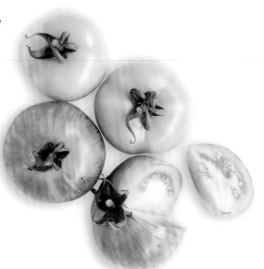

What neither study mentioned is that heirloom toms like Green Zebra, which keep their verdant stripes even when ripe, are some of the tastiest around. With unripe tomatoes – delicious fried, in salsas and simmered into chutneys – I am all about upping my dose, while I wait for more solid evidence to come in.

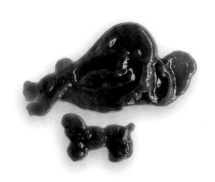

☕ THE SECRET'S IN THE SAUCE (OR CAN)

Lycopene may have intriguing health benefits but it does have one big downfall: it isn't very easy for our bodies to absorb. Trapped deep within the tomato cells, lycopene is hard to get at – well, until tomatoes are cooked, that is.

Ever notice how cooked tomatoes in soups, sauces and casseroles (whatever, really) almost indelibly stain plastic storage containers, but chopped fresh tomatoes don't? This is because as little as 30 minutes bubbling on the stove can more than double the amount of bright red lycopene available in the fruit. Heat not only breaks open the cells releasing the pigment, it also transforms the lycopene molecules from hard-to-absorb crystals to a much more soluble form that is easier for your body to get at almost as if by magic. Yes, cooked tomatoes – and that includes canned ones – are much better for you than raw ones, at least in terms of their lycopene content. This is just as well, considering almost 60 per cent of those consumed in countries like the USA are in the cheaper and more convenient canned form.

The richest form of all is concentrated tomato purée, which isn't just cooked, but reduced down by evaporating off some of its water, making a product that is a whopping 16 times richer in lycopene than the same volume of fresh tomatoes, according to the USDA.

ROASTED CHERRY TOMATO SAUCE

This is probably the simplest tomato sauce recipe known to man. No tomato peeling, chopping, sautéing or simmering involved, just pure knock-out flavour. Roasting tomatoes causes them to lose water, concentrating the chemicals within the fruit, creating a sauce with richer flavour and enhanced nutrition. Using unpeeled cherry tomatoes adds to the total lycopene content of the dish (not to mention saving you the faff), and a drizzle of extra virgin olive oil to finish helps you absorb even more of the good stuff.

MAKES 1KG
PREP TIME 10 MINUTES
COOK TIME 40 MINUTES

1KG CHERRY TOMATOES
1 LARGE ONION, SLICED
2 GARLIC CLOVES, PEELED AND LEFT WHOLE
4 TBSP EXTRA VIRGIN OLIVE OIL
1 TSP RED CHILLI FLAKES
1 TBSP BALSAMIC VINEGAR
100G TOASTED FLAKED ALMONDS
½ TSP SALT
½ TSP BLACK PEPPER
SMALL HANDFUL OF BASIL LEAVES, TORN

PREHEAT the oven to 200°C/Gas Mark 6.

TOSS together all the ingredients except the basil in a roasting tin and roast for 40 minutes.

STIR the basil through the tomatoes to combine.

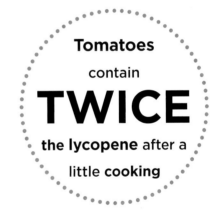

Tomatoes contain **TWICE** the lycopene after a little cooking

HOW TO SERVE

This Roasted Cherry Tomato Sauce is as versatile as it is easy to make. It freezes beautifully, too, making it a handy standby for super-fast healthy food.
Here are a few ideas to get you started...

1 BRUSCHETTA

Toast 4 large slices of **wholemeal sourdough bread** and drizzle with a little **extra virgin olive oil**. Scatter over a handful of **rocket leaves**, then divide 250g **Roasted Cherry Tomato Sauce** among the toasts and serve.

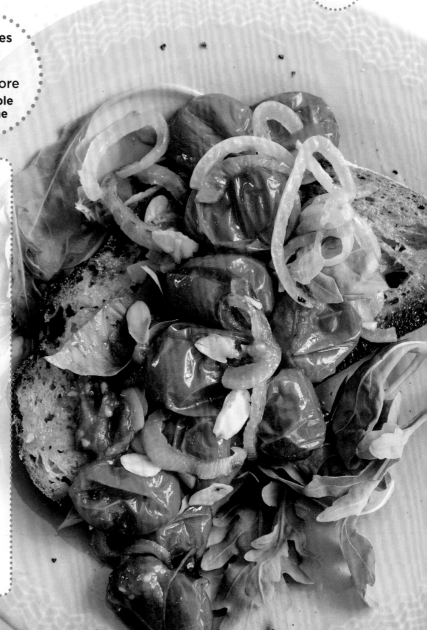

1

Tomatoes + oil =

3Xmore absorbable lycopene

SPLASH ON THE OIL

Scientists at Deakin University, Australia, found that by simply adding 1 tablespoon of olive oil per 300g of cooked toms, the amount of easy-to-absorb soluble lycopene in participants' blood shot up to almost three times that of those eating the exact same quantity of tomatoes without the oil.

But it's not just the lycopene that benefits from the added fat. A team from the University of Barcelona found that enriching tomato sauce with olive oil also boosted the absorption of potentially heart-healthy chemicals called polyphenols. This splash of oil not only improved nutrient absorption (making it what the geeks call 'more bioavailable'), it also had a measurable effect on the ability of the sauce to reduce the risk factors of cardiovascular disease in the participants who consumed it, significantly outdoing that of fat-free sauces. Don't like olive oil? Well, it appears other fats may work just as well. Add some avocado to salsa and it can quadruple how much lycopene you absorb, according to the Ohio State University.

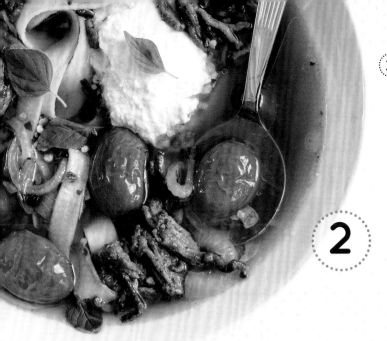

2 LASAGNE SOUP

Heat 1 tsp **olive oil** in a saucepan and fry 200g **minced beef** until browned. Add 8 **fresh lasagne sheets**, sliced into strips, 1 **bay leaf**, 1 tbsp **tomato purée**, 1 litre hot **beef stock** and 200g **Roasted Cherry Tomato Sauce** and simmer for 10 minutes until the pasta is tender and the beef cooked through. Ladle into 4 bowls and serve each topped with 1 tbsp **fresh ricotta cheese** and a sprinkling of **red chilli flakes** and **oregano leaves or flowers.**

2

GRATE ON THE CHEESE

Just as with olive oil, tomatoes and cheese are a match made in culinary heaven. It's great news then that a study by the *Journal of Nutrition* found that consuming tomato extracts with milk protein also significantly boosted the bioavailability of the lycopene they contained, even more so than concentrated tomato purée – the richest source currently known.

OK, so the study was conducted at the Nestlé Research Centre, which is also responsible for marketing the now-patented formula, but it does reflect results from similar studies on milk potentially being a good delivery mechanism for other related carotene pigments. Either way, it's a welcome excuse to add a grating of Parmesan, a spoonful of ricotta or a crumbling of feta to every tomato dish I make. Why not?

3

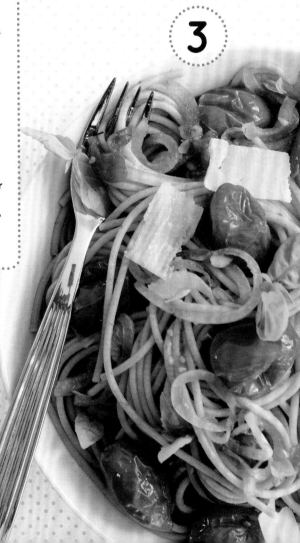

3 CHERRY TOMATO PASTA

Spoon some **Roasted Cherry Tomato Sauce** over hot **pasta**, add a generous sprinkling of **Parmesan cheese** shavings and some **basil leaves** and serve.

SALAD LEAVES

Calorie for calorie, leafy greens are officially some of the most nutrient dense of all fruit and veg, at least according to the US government's Centers for Disease Control and Prevention. In its ranking of foods that provide the highest concentrations of 17 key nutrients essential for human health, every entry in the top ten is greens. Leafy greens also possess a range of phytonutrients that have been shown in some studies to inhibit the growth of certain types of cancer (in test tubes, at least). If all the above wasn't enough, here are two more things they might do for you…

MANAGING WEIGHT

I am often asked if there is some miraculous plant that can help you to lose weight. My answer has always been, 'If there was, I'd be a good ten pounds lighter and about a million pounds richer.' But, if any commonly eaten food comes close to having 'negative calories', leafy greens are it, at least that's what a study published in the *Journal of the American Dietetic Association* seems to suggest.

Give volunteers a large leafy salad as a first course before a carb-tastic buffet of pasta, where they can eat as much as they want, and guess what? They eat less – in fact, up to 12 per cent less. Even once the caloric value of the salad was taken into account, the total calorie content of the meal was slashed by as much as 100 calories. But it doesn't have to be a starter, either; almost identical findings have been reported by a similar but totally unrelated trial at Pennsylvania State University, which served the salad with the main course.

Ladies and gentlemen, I give you 'negative calories' – well, sort of. If you go wild with high-fat dressings and cheese the effects are cancelled out, but to me there has never been a better reason to add a crisp green salad to a meal.

CARDIO HEALTH

A team at the University of Toronto added 250g of frozen spinach to some chicken broth with a bit of onion and pepper to make a simple soup and fed it to an (admittedly very small) group of volunteers each day. The researchers found the soup eaters' blood pressure was significantly reduced and their arteries became less stiff after just 7 days, according to this preliminary study. The authors attributed this to the dietary nitrate found in spinach. What are the richest food sources of this promising chemical? Aside from red beetroot (see page 83), it's greens – especially rocket, spinach, lettuce, cress and celery.

(DARK) GREEN MEANS 'GO'

We tend to talk about leafy greens as a whole, like they are one generic type of veg. However, in reality they are a collection of loads of completely unrelated species that just happen to have edible leaves, meaning their chemical contents, and therefore nutritional value, can vary enormously between types. And the wonderful thing about plant science is once you understand why plants produce these chemicals, there are super-easy visual cues to where the goodness lies.

Dark leafy veg like kale, spinach, watercress and even the deeper green lettuce varieties generally contain significantly more vitamins, minerals and other phytonutrients than their paler cousins. How much more? Well, here are some stats for you. Pick darker green Romaine lettuce over pallid Iceberg and for starters you'd get up to an astonishing 20 times the vitamin A and antioxidant betacarotene, according to Colorado State University. But the benefits don't end there. When it comes to folic acid and vitamin K, the Colorado team found you'd have to eat five servings of Iceberg just to get the same amount as a single serving of Romaine. In fact, any darker-leaved lettuce they studied turned out to be higher in every major vitamin, mineral and phytonutrient, without exception, than light green Iceberg.

This is because of the role colour plays in plant leaves. Dark green leafy veg are packed with a group of antioxidant pigments called carotenes, which give many orange fruit and veg like pumpkins, sweet potatoes and, of course, carrots their characteristic golden hue. One of their functions in leaves is to act as a sort of natural sunscreen, mopping up harmful free radicals, helping protect cells from damage. When we eat these chemicals, their protective antioxidant effects can be transferred to our own cells, with studies suggesting they can prevent DNA damage that may lead to cancer and even shield our eyes from the UV damage that can lead to age-related sight loss. Some of these carotenes can even be converted by our bodies to make vitamin A too.

In fact, dark green leafy veg like kale can, surprisingly, contain more of these orange carotene pigments than even vivid golden veg like pumpkins. How is this possible? Well, it's just that their yellow and orange tones are masked by the light green chlorophyll pigments also found in leaves, creating their darker hue. The more carotenes a leaf contains, the darker green it appears. That explains why although mid-green Romaine lettuce might have twenty times the levels of some carotenes than light-coloured Iceberg, the super-dark leaves of kale boast a whopping 52 times the amount. That's before we even mention it also has 30 times the vitamin K and 40 times the vitamin C.

🧺 LOOSE LEAVES, GAIN NUTRITION

Another reason why lettuce varieties like Romaine contain more nutrients than Iceberg is the very structure of how their leaves are arranged. Weird, I know. We have spent hundreds of years breeding leafy crops like lettuce, cabbages and endive to form tightly closed heads of densely wrapped foliage instead of the open, airy structure that these plants have in the wild, where the leaves bask facing the sun. Protected within a ball-like head, the leaves are not exposed to the harsh UV light, battering winds and predation from insects and therefore don't produce the tough fibres and bitter defence chemicals they normally would need. The shame here is that these are the exact same chemicals that provide these crops with many of their nutritional benefits.

The stark difference between sun-exposed leaves and those that are shaded deep within the heart was recently shown in a study in the *Journal of Food Biochemistry*. The authors found that on the same lettuce plant the external leaves could contain twice the antioxidant activity, three times the heart-healthy polyphenols and a whopping five times the carotenes than those in the centre. Seemingly without exception, loose-leafed varieties of leafy greens, whose leaves grow exposed to the sun, will contain far more phytonutrients than tightly closed ones.

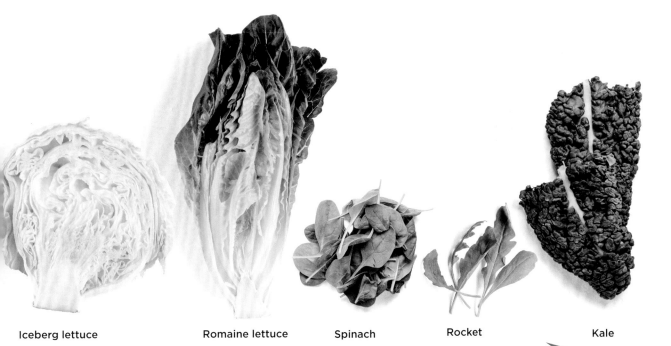

Iceberg lettuce   Romaine lettuce   Spinach   Rocket   Kale

FEWER NUTRIENTS   **MORE NUTRIENTS**

Compared to Iceberg lettuce...

Romaine lettuce has
• **20x** the vitamin A
• **5x** the vitamin K
• **5x** the folic acid

Kale has
• **52x** the carotenes
• **40x** the vitamin C
• **30x** the Vitamin K

THE REDDER THE BETTER

If leafy greens are good for you, leafy 'reds' might be even better and again it's the pigments at work. Many plants produce red and purple pigments called anthocyanins as antioxidant defences to help further protect their new growth against UV damage. These happen to be the same group of compounds that give many 'superfood' fruit like blueberries and black grapes their characteristic colour. Because we find them instinctively attractive, many leafy crops have been bred to accentuate this feature, resulting in deep purple cabbages (see page 35), claret-coloured chicories and Lollo Rossa lettuce, splattered with burgundy tones.

Not only do they look beautiful on your plate but these coloured veg also come with significantly higher phytonutrient content as a result. Go for red radicchio instead of pale curly endive and you get up to five times more polyphenols – that's almost 50 per cent more than polyphenol-packed dark green spinach. Likewise, compare purple-tinged Lollo Rossa with bright green Romaine and you get over 20 times the polyphenols. And next to Iceberg? There is an almost unbelievable 690-fold leap in polyphenol content between the deepest red over the very palest green.

What a shame therefore that pallid Iceberg lettuce is the fifth most popular vegetable in the US diet (which is increasingly reflective of global food culture), where it is by far the most commonly eaten leafy green. Consumed to this level, making a simple switch to darker greens could start to add up, over time potentially making a noticeable impact on vitamin, mineral and phytonutrient intake, and yet be barely noticeable in terms of texture and flavour.

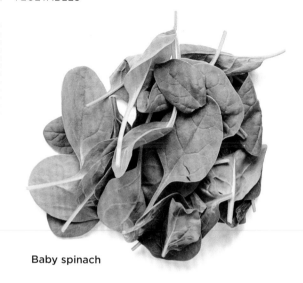

Baby spinach

BIG VS BABY LEAVES

Love those handy 'washed and ready-to-eat' supermarket packets of baby leaves? Well, when it comes to spinach, they might just be a healthier choice, too. According to the Swedish University of Agricultural Sciences, baby spinach leaves had significantly more polyphenols when compared to those harvested at a mature stage, with the researchers concluding that by picking them at this younger stage the nutrient 'concentration in the product may be increased and the content of potentially health-promoting compounds enhanced'. The same principle is likely to be the case for the closely related baby chard and beet leaves too.

However, leafy greens in the crucifer family like kale, cabbage and pak choi have been shown to have a directly opposite tendency across a range of studies, accumulating nutrients as they grow – containing up to double the levels of key phytonutrients called glucosinolates (see page 34) of the young plants. The moral of the story? For spinach, beets and chard, baby leaves are a great choice; for pretty much everything else, go for the big boys.

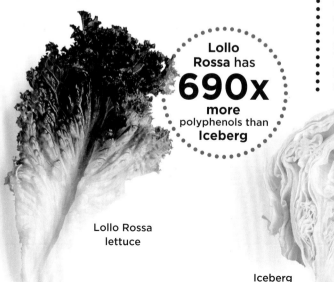

Lollo
Rossa has
690x
more
polyphenols than
Iceberg

**Lollo Rossa
lettuce**

**Iceberg
lettuce**

🥗 LOVE BAGGED SALAD

I am forever reading scare stories in the press about how bad for you bagged salad is, yet research shows that typical harvesting and storage of salad crops have little effect on their vitamin and polyphenol content – in one Spanish study of nine different baby-leaf salads, for example, there was little appreciable difference after 10 days storage, apart from a decline in vitamin C. In mature leaves of kale, harvested samples held in refrigerated commercial storage for an astonishing 6 weeks showed no change in antioxidant activity when compared to live plants still in the field, again apart from a dent in the vitamin C levels. Add a spritz of vitamin C-rich lemon juice to your salad dressing and this dip is soon cancelled out (see 'Dress Them Up', right), making super-convenient bagged salad a great choice.

🥗 TREAT IT MEAN, KEEP IT KEEN

There is one simple thing you can do to your veg in storage to positively send its phytonutrient levels soaring: wound it. You see, many of the protective antioxidant compounds in leaves are generated at the sites of injury, helping shield their tissues from further damage – in a process food scientists call 'wounding'. To non-geeks this is also known as slicing or tearing, just as you would do when preparing a salad. Pop cut lettuce or leafy endive in a sealed container (or plastic food bag) in the fridge overnight to give these chemical reactions time to happen and their polyphenol levels can jump up 50 per cent,

according to the University of Pisa in Italy. OK, so these leaves do start to decline after they peak, but even after 3 days they still contained more good stuff than they started out with. Hurrah for leftovers and packed lunches!

♨ DRESS THEM UP

Eating your greens doesn't have to mean tucking into a spartan plate of raw foliage; in fact, studies have shown that adding creamy dressings or sautéing them up into tasty dishes positively increases their many benefits. Here's how to boost their nutritional value and flavour at the same time.

Remember those ghastly fat-free bottled dressings of the 90s? Some things are best left in the past, especially as oil has since been shown to be essential for the absorption of fat-soluble nutrients like carotenes and vitamins A and K in leafy greens. In one trial by the *American Journal of Clinical Nutrition*, researchers found that volunteers eating a salad of spinach, Romaine lettuce, cherry tomatoes and carrots surprisingly showed zero absorption of these key compounds when served with a fat-free dressing. Essentially, none whatsoever, despite each of the ingredients being excellent sources of a range of different carotenes. Serve the exact same salad with a half-fat dressing and their absorption was significantly improved, but nowhere near as much as when it was served with a creamy, full-fat one. Yeh!

It appears that it is not just the amount of fat but the *type* of fat that can make a huge difference. According to the journal *Molecular Nutrition & Food Research*, monounsaturated fats enhance the absorption of these phytonutrients far more effectively than saturated or polyunsaturated fats. A classic olive oil dressing is a great source of monounsaturated fats, as is a handful of crunchy nuts tossed through the salad, or half a creamy avocado sliced over the top. Speaking of avocados, one trial at the Ohio State University found that adding about one sliced avo to a salad could boost the absorption of antioxidant betacarotene an astonishing 15-fold, and other carotenes like lutein and zeaxanthin (which may protect ageing eyes) up to five times more.

Add a squirt of vitamin C-rich lemon juice to that dressing and you could improve the iron in leafy greens like spinach and watercress up to three times, according to the *American Journal of Clinical Nutrition*. Mix olive oil and lemon together to make a simple dressing and you could vastly improve the flavour and nutrition benefits of any salad. And guess what? I have recipes for a fresh mustardy one and a creamy ranch-style one for that very reason (see pages 41 and 166).

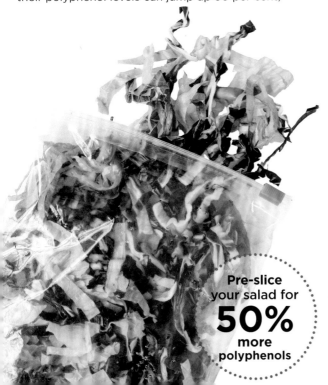

Pre-slice your salad for **50%** more polyphenols

☕ COOK UP SOME NUTRITION

You might be forgiven for thinking that eating leafy greens raw is the best way to access their nutrition. After all fresh, crisp leaves are in their most natural state possible, and there is a whole 'raw food movement' with thousands of online devotees espousing the many benefits of uncooked veg. However, a stack of studies has consistently shown that light cooking not only doesn't damage the nutritional content of greens, but can also greatly improve it. Heat application breaks open the cells in these leaves, releasing the nutrients they contain, thereby allowing them to be better absorbed. You can even see this process in action when cooked greens become significantly 'greener' after just a few minutes of steaming, sautéing or microwaving. How much more? Well, in one trial, blood tests on women eating cooked spinach for 3 weeks revealed levels of carotenes three times higher than those eating the same amount of spinach in raw form. From just a practical point of view, anyone who has ever cooked spinach will know that a giant packet of the fresh stuff cooks down to only a couple of tablespoons. I tested this at home and found that five large portions of the raw leaves turned into just one small portion of the cooked stuff after less than a minute in a hot pan – meaning not only did the veg contain more available nutrition but I could eat far more of it. Two portions of the cooked stuff made a tasty side dish – if it was raw it would have made enough salad to cover every surface in my kitchen. I like salad, but not that much.

There are some ways of cooking greens that appear to be much better at conserving their ingredients than others. Steam or microwave kale and its antioxidant and polyphenol levels jump 40 per cent, for example; boil it and about half of these leach into the cooking water. Fine if you are making a soup or stew in which you consume this liquid; a bit of a wasted exercise, though, if this is destined to be tipped down the sink. For a range of other greens it seems the same holds true, so stick to light steaming, sautéing and microwaving, but leave boiling for soups and stews.

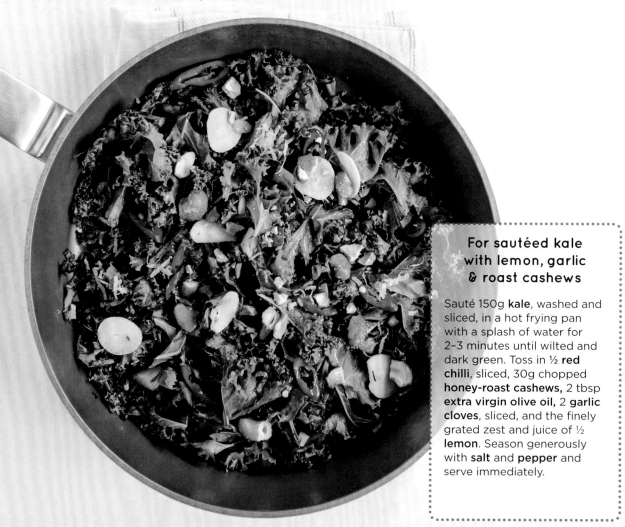

For sautéed kale with lemon, garlic & roast cashews

Sauté 150g **kale**, washed and sliced, in a hot frying pan with a splash of water for 2–3 minutes until wilted and dark green. Toss in ½ **red chilli**, sliced, 30g chopped **honey-roast cashews**, 2 tbsp **extra virgin olive oil**, 2 **garlic cloves**, sliced, and the finely grated zest and juice of ½ **lemon**. Season generously with **salt** and **pepper** and serve immediately.

SALAD BY STEALTH

The grown-up bitterness of veg like kale or radicchio can be a tricky sell to kids. Paired with the sweetness of fruit and blitzed up into colourful smoothies, however, they become totally undetectable, meaning even the most dedicated little sugar monsters can love greens (just make the smoothies while their backs are turned). Simply blitz together all the ingredients listed for either smoothie in a blender or food processor until smooth, pour into a glass and serve straight away.

KIWI & MANGO SMOOTHIE
(with hidden spinach)

'No darling, the green comes from kiwis...': a white lie any unsuspecting veg phobic will believe. The fat in the almonds aids the absorption of the carotenoids, while adding a wonderful creaminess.

Small handful of baby spinach leaves + 1 unpeeled gold kiwifruit + ½ peeled and stoned mango + 1 wedge of lemon + 10 whole almonds + 250ml water + natural stevia sweetener, to taste (optional)

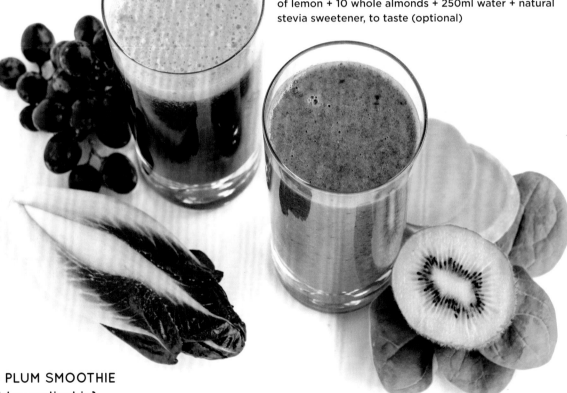

GRAPE & PLUM SMOOTHIE
(with hidden radicchio)

Salad smoothies don't have to be green either! Red leaves are great at hiding incognito between dark fruit like grapes and plums.

Small handful of radicchio leaves + handful of black grapes + 1 stoned and roughly chopped black plum + ½ mandarin + 250 ml water + natural stevia sweetener, to taste (optional)

THE CABBAGE FAMILY

Just like other leafy greens, the veg in the cabbage family (called 'crucifers' in geek speak) are real nutritional superstars, providing calorie for calorie more essential nutrients like vitamins A, C and folic acid than pretty much any other fruit or veg. But why make a section dedicated to them alone? Well, it's the growing body of research pointing to the potential for a group of chemicals uniquely found in this veg family to prevent degenerative diseases that did it. Science may still be piecing the puzzle together, but here's the latest.

♡ CRUCIFERS AGAINST CANCER?

In order to fight back against attack from insect predators these plants have evolved the ability to generate pungent, bitter-tasting, sulphur-based compounds called glucosinolates. When chopped, chewed or digested, glucosinolates break down into substances called isothiocyanates, which possess interesting biological effects. While these might be acutely toxic to tiny insects, in our, much bigger, bodies they paradoxically may have a protective effect according to a growing stack of research. Test-tube and animal studies have shown that glucosinolates and their products can suppress cancer cell development in the colon, lungs, liver, bladder, breast and stomach, and research looking at dietary patterns has frequently (but by no means always) shown that people who eat more of these vegetables tend to have a statistically lower risk of developing certain cancers.

The crazy thing about the products of glucosinolates is that they appear to work in at least three totally different ways. Not only do they demonstrate the ability in some test-tube and animal studies to stop cancer cells from multiplying and even to naturally self-destruct, while ignoring healthy cells, they also appear to be able to neutralize cell-damaging free radicals that are associated with developing cancer in the first place. Other studies have suggested they may go even further, triggering your body's own natural defences against carcinogenic substances by stimulating the secretion of enzymes that mop these up before they have a chance to damage cells. This suggests a theoretical trifecta of cell defence, attacking from all sides, *if* these studies are replicable in humans.

The effects of glucosinolate consumption can start to be seen pretty quickly, too. In one Italian study, by adding 3 servings of broccoli (that's a lot of broccoli!) to the daily diets of male smokers, a significant reduction in the inflammation associated with several degenerative diseases was seen in as little as 10 days. In another small trial funded by the US-based National Cancer Institute, adding about 150g of various cruciferous veg to participants' daily diets was able to reduce levels of oxidative stress (a risk factor for developing certain cancers) by an impressive 22 per cent in just 3 weeks.

OK, so these trials were both very small and extremely short term, and it is important to point out that other human studies have shown mixed results. More evidence is clearly needed before any hard and fast conclusions are drawn, but there does appear to be a growing body of research that suggests that adding a couple of servings of this group of veg to your daily diet could be a particularly healthy choice. This section will show you how to get the best from them.

🧺 SELECTING THE BEST OF THE BEST

Despite looking almost unrecognizably different, most crops in the cabbage family – including everything from turnips to cauliflower, mustard to red cabbage – are incredibly closely related. In fact, every vegetable on the opposite page technically belongs to just one species, bred to create myriad forms and flavours by thousands of years of farmers selecting for different traits. This is also reflected in their internal chemistry, meaning that when it comes to glucosinolates some varieties can contain almost 20 times more than others gram for gram. Thanks to a couple of supergeeks at the University of Queensland, who pooled the findings of more than 18 studies, we now have a really reliable ranking of the best of the best. So here goes...

Brussels sprouts have **5x** the potentially **cancer-fighting glucosinolates** of even extremely close relatives like **cauliflower**

Brussels sprouts

With nearly five times the glucosinolates of close relatives like cauliflower these guys provide the most glucosinolate bang for buck. Closely followed by spring greens (200mg/100g), these two veg leave the others in the dust.

Savoy cabbage

The humble Savoy might be a runner-up in the glucosinolate stakes with less than half that of Brussels sprouts, but compared to other cabbages it is far richer.

Kale

Kale has a similar glucosinolate level to Savoy cabbage, but there is so much more to nutritional value than fixating on a single compound. Containing many times more vitamins A, C and K than any of the other crops on this page, kale is by no means an inferior choice. When it comes to polyphenols, it has more than twice that of Brussels sprouts, too, so enjoy both liberally.

White & red cabbages

White and red cabbage contain about 40 per cent less glucosinolates than Savoy cabbage. What red cabbage lacks in glucosinolates however it more than makes up for in polyphenol content, with several trials consistently ranking it as the highest of all cabbages in these potentially heart-healthy compounds, owing to the rich anthocyanin content.

What about white cabbage? Sadly this guy loses out in both stakes, containing less than half the polyphenols of red, which has between two and five times the antioxidant activity of its white cousin. Another reminder that dark green or red leafy veg are generally more nutrient dense than their paler cousins.

Broccoli

Well, here's a surprising one. Broccoli, the cabbage family's pin-up for health benefits, actually ranks relatively low in terms of total glucosinolates. But it is the *type* of glucosinolates it contains that has sparked the interest, as it is by far the richest in a specific one called glucoraphanin, which research suggests may be particularly beneficial (see 'Super Broccoli!', page 36). It is also one of the highest of all crucifers in heart-healthy polyphenols, alongside kale.

Cauliflower

Last, and sadly kind of least, comes the humble cauliflower. Containing just 80 per cent fewer glucosinolates than Brussels sprouts and just half the polyphenols of broccoli, this guy isn't a clear winner in the nutrition stakes.

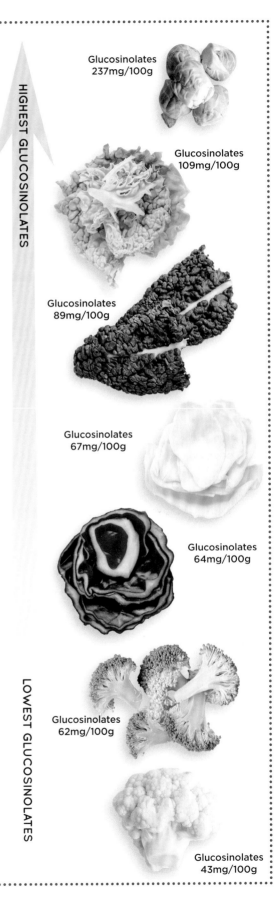

HIGHEST GLUCOSINOLATES

LOWEST GLUCOSINOLATES

Glucosinolates 237mg/100g

Glucosinolates 109mg/100g

Glucosinolates 89mg/100g

Glucosinolates 67mg/100g

Glucosinolates 64mg/100g

Glucosinolates 62mg/100g

Glucosinolates 43mg/100g

🧺 SUPER BROCCOLI!

Of all the different types of glucosinolates (there are over 100), the one that has traditionally attracted the most interest from researchers is a compound found almost exclusively in broccoli called glucoraphanin.

In animal trials this has been associated with reducing the risk of everything from cancer to heart disease and diabetes – the big killers of modern times. But would this translate to humans? A team of Brazilian researchers pooled together the results of over a dozen of the best-quality recent clinical trials from around the world that aimed to answer just that question by adding glucoraphanin to people's diets and measuring the effects. They found that while there was less solid evidence for cancer protection, there was a more consistent pattern in the evidence to suggest that adding glucoraphanin to the diet may help lower cholesterol, control blood sugar and reduce oxidative stress. This is some of the strongest evidence we have so far for the potential health benefits associated with broccoli consumption. However, as always, picking the right variety can make a big difference.

Research has consistently shown that sprouting broccoli varieties are more phytonutrient dense than traditional round heads, with up to three times the total glucosinolates, twice as many polyphenols and loads more vitamin C. With their added purple anthocyanin pigments, purple sprouting ones are likely to have even more of an antioxidant edge.

Want to go one better? There is a new British conventional broccoli variety that has been bred by crossing traditional cultivars with the plant's wild relatives in southern Italy to create a sort of naturally supercharged broccoli that produces a whopping two to three times more of the specific glucosinolate, glucoraphanin, attributed with broccoli's benefits than the regular kind, while maintaining the same high levels of all other nutrients. Marketed under the glossy name 'Beneforté', it appeared to be three times more effective than the regular stuff at reducing 'bad' LDL cholesterol in small, short-term clinical trials.

🍳 THE FRESHER THE BETTER

Broccoli is one of those veg you should get scoffing as soon as you can. This is because as soon as it is harvested the florets experience a precipitous decline of nutritional value. A Spanish research team aimed to replicate the conditions that broccoli is typically subjected to from field to fork – storing it at 1°C for a week to mimic industrial transport and storage, followed by 3 days at 15°C to simulate it sitting on the store shelves – with some brow-raising results. By the time broccoli gets to you it could have lost 80 per cent of its glucosinolates. These findings were echoed by others. One study in the journal *Food Chemistry* found that broccoli could lose up to 70 per cent of its vitamin C and betacarotene and 50 per cent of its antioxidant activity in just 6 days. Yikes!

Fortunately, there is a simple solution that involves no extra work for you. The same research also showed that keeping the broccoli continuously refrigerated and stored in sealed bags (as opposed to unwrapped in the fridge) could stem these declines almost entirely. The take-home? Only buy broccoli in sealed bags from the chiller cabinet, not loose on the shelves, pick bags with the longest possible expiry date and cook and eat it as soon as you can. Done.

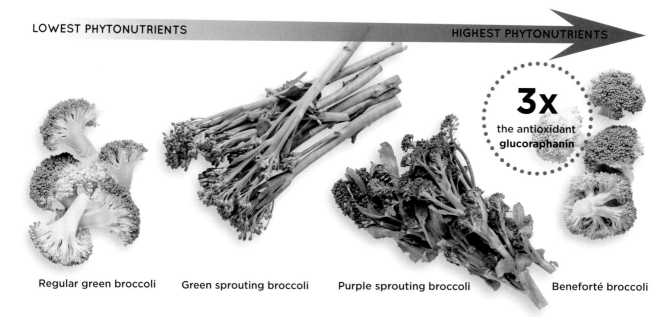

LOWEST PHYTONUTRIENTS → HIGHEST PHYTONUTRIENTS

3x the antioxidant glucoraphanin

Regular green broccoli   Green sprouting broccoli   Purple sprouting broccoli   Beneforté broccoli

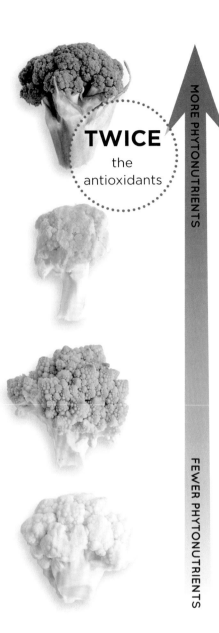

TWICE
the antioxidants

MORE PHYTONUTRIENTS

FEWER PHYTONUTRIENTS

▭ TECHNI-CAULIFLOWER

Cauliflower might be the poor relative of the crucifer family when it comes to, well, pretty much every nutrient. Compare it with kale, for example, which has twice the vitamin C, five times the polyphenols and a whopping 67 times the carotenes. However, there is a simple trick to massively increase its nutritional content and that is to pick any variety that isn't white.

Purple

The crazy psychedelic curds of purple cauliflower were recently found by the Norwegian University of Life Sciences to have twice the polyphenols and antioxidant activity of a range of white and green forms (orange was not included in the trial, so we don't know how the two compare). They also have a sweeter, less bitter taste than the white, holding on well to their colour as long as you cook them right. The purple pigments are highly water soluble so boiling or blanching will mean loads of these just leach into the cooking water. If steamed, sautéed or roasted, however, purple cauli will maintain all its lavender glory, especially if spritzed with lemon juice beforehand. Pickled, the curds are a beauty to behold.

Orange

Go for one of the bright orange caulis and you could get 25 times more vitamin A than the white stuff. It retains its colour brilliantly, too, so you can cook it in all the ways you would the regular kind.

Green

Pick a weirdly fractal-shaped green cauli, which I find have a far richer flavour with a delicious nuttiness to them, and you instantly bump up the vitamin C content a third and get 20 per cent more polyphenols over white according to the Norwegians.

White

This is essentially a coloured cauliflower with all the nutritious pigments stripped out, creating a white canvas – both visually and nutritionally. Still a healthy veg, just nowhere near as much as the others.

STEAM, SAUTÉ OR MICROWAVE

Steaming crucifers
retains **2x** the **antioxidants** compared to boiling

Loads of studies have looked at the nutritional impact cooking has on cruciferous veg and have consistently found that the method you choose to serve them can have a really important impact on the nutritional content of the resultant dish.

STEAM, SAUTÉ OR MICROWAVE crucifers with minimum amount of water and you can increase their levels of vitamin A and antioxidant carotenes up to five times by breaking open cells, allowing these nutrients to be released. Adding a splash of oil in the process makes these even more easy for your body to absorb.

BOIL them, however, and more than half of their total antioxidant activity can be destroyed along with heart-healthy polyphenols and vitamin C. The longer you do this for the worse it gets.

RED CABBAGE & APPLE SLAW

Swap palid white cabbage for the brilliant purple kind when you make slaw and not only do you get a more vibrant plate of food, but also a whopping ten times the vitamin A, twice the iron and double the antioxidants. Slaw doesn't have to mean a grease-fest either. This deliciously fresh recipe teams up red cabbage with red onions for a double anthocyanin dose for your next cook-off. Halfway between a crisp salad and a tangy condiment, it works just as well with BBQ chicken and corn as it does roast pork and mash in the winter.

SERVES 4

PREP TIME 10 MINUTES,
PLUS INFUSING

....

200G RED CABBAGE, FINELY SHREDDED

1 CARROT, GRATED

1 RED CHILLI, FINELY SHREDDED

½ RED ONION, FINELY SHREDDED

1 GREEN APPLE, FINELY SHREDDED

½ TSP SALT

FINELY GRATED ZEST AND JUICE OF 1 LIME

1 TSP OLIVE OIL

1 TSP SUGAR

TOSS all the ingredients together in a large mixing bowl with your hands to ensure everything is evenly mixed. Continue to massage the mixture, squeezing it between your fingers until it starts to slightly soften.

COVER and leave to infuse in the fridge for 30 minutes.

SLICE IT FINE

Slicing and dicing cruciferous veg does more than just make it easier to cook and eat – it amazingly is actually capable of triggering off all sorts of complex chemical reactions in the raw veg, which can make it measurably better for you. Sound too good to be true? Let me explain. Even once harvested, veg are still living plants, and they react to this simulated pest damage by attempting to defend themselves. Once their cells are broken open an enzyme called myrosinase reacts with the glucosinolates like a chemical flare to kick out compounds called isothiocyanates. It is actually these protective isothiocyanates that we believe to be what's really behind many of the crucifers' health benefits. The glucosinolates only matter because of what they turn into. The finer you chop crucifers, the more of this reaction takes place and the more isothiocyanate benefit you are likely to get. This reaction, of course, also happens when you chew the raw veg; however, by finely chopping the veg and leaving it for an hour or two before eating (or cooking) it there is a greater amount of time for this reaction to take place – potentially giving you even more of the good stuff.

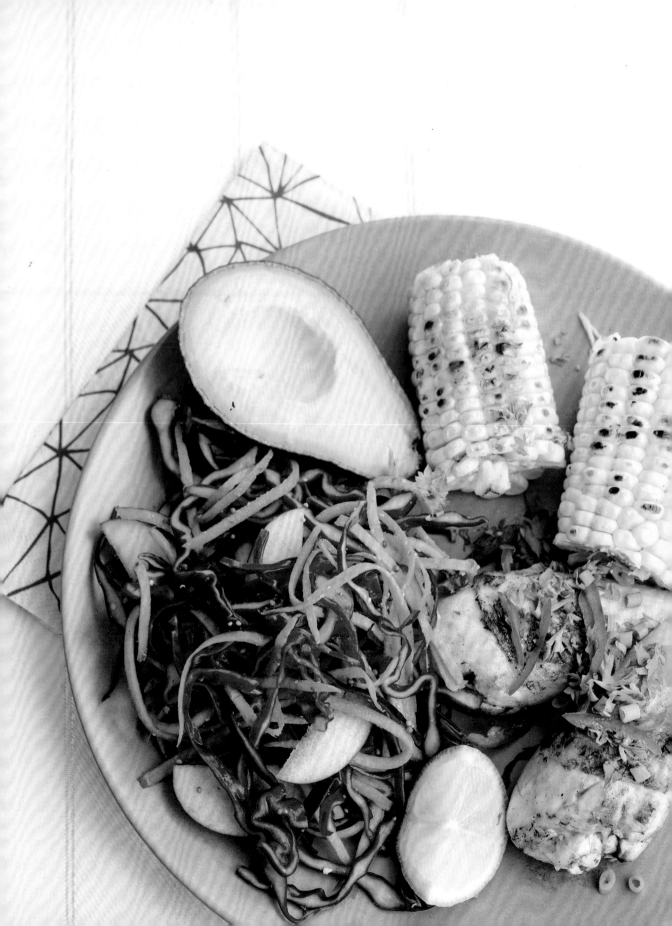

'MAGIC MUSTARD' DRESSING

What you serve with cooked crucifers can have a truly phenomenal impact on their potential health benefits, even greater than that of variety choice, and it's all to do with a little bit of kitchen chemistry. You see, despite crucifers having loads of glucosinolates, it's really a separate group of chemicals called isothiocyanates that these break down into that actually appears to hold the health promise (see my chemical flare analogy on page 38). The fierce heat of cooking, however, stops the production of these all-important isothiocyanates dead in its tracks, by destroying the enzyme that is responsible for the chemical reaction. Damn! In fact, one Dutch study found that cooking broccoli could slash the absorbable isothiocyanate levels a whopping 90 per cent, and the exact same effect appears in other cruciferous veg too.

Fortunately, food science has come to the rescue in the form of a team from the University of Reading who found that simply adding a tiny amount of powdered mustard seeds (also a cruciferous plant, which contains a heat-resistant form of the enzyme) to cooked crucifers like broccoli restores their ability to generate the isothiocyanate. Adding just half a teaspoon of mustard powder for every 200g of cooked crucifers made them, almost as if by magic, pretty much as good as raw.

The best bit? Mustard is a natural flavour enhancer so your veg actually tastes better as a result. This mustard dressing – based on Reading Uni's calculations – is all you need to transform the average 300g head of broccoli.

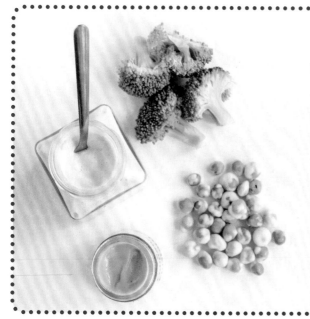

DON'T LIKE MUSTARD?

The same enzyme is also found in loads of other condiments like horseradish, wasabi and, of course, wasabi peas, which add a lovely crunch scattered over a bowl of greens. You can even mix raw and cooked cruciferous veg and the reaction still works. Researchers trying to figure out how to make microwaveable packs of frozen broccoli more nutritious found that adding a tiny amount of raw radish had a similar effect. So why not chuck a handful of rocket, watercress or even shredded raw sprouts or red cabbage (all also cruciferous veg) into your next crucifer sauté just as it hits the table for added flavour and phytonutrients? Mustard haters rejoice!

MAKES ENOUGH TO SERVE WITH
1 HEAD OF COOKED BROCCOLI

PREP TIME 5 MINUTES

2 TBSP EXTRA VIRGIN OLIVE OIL

2 TSP LEMON JUICE

1 TSP MUSTARD POWDER

LARGE PINCH OF SEA SALT

¼ TSP DRIED DILL

¼ TSP CLEAR HONEY

WHISK all the ingredients together in a bowl.

USE immediately. If you make larger batches of this dressing, it can be stored in a sealed jar in the fridge for up to 2 weeks.

Broccoli, made better

Serving cooked broccoli with raw cruciferous veg like **rocket** or **watercress** can have a similar effect to mustard, so why not add both? Chuck in some **pistachios** and crumbled **feta cheese**, and that's the veg course sorted.

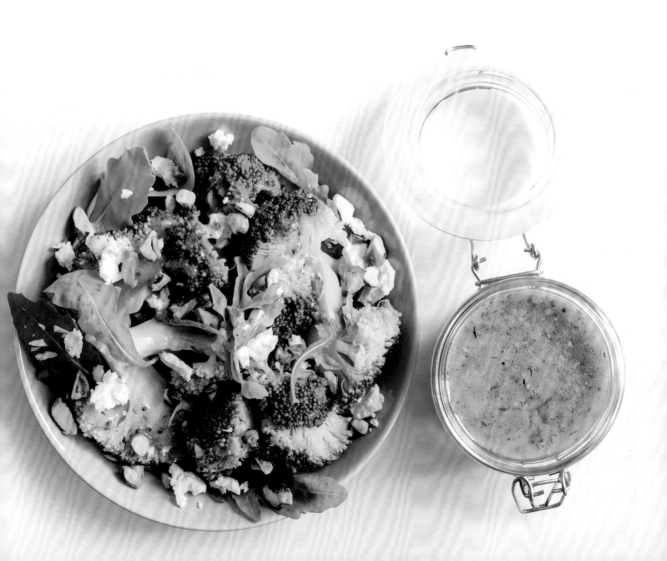

RAW BROCCOLI & ALMOND PESTO

OK, so we know that one of the healthiest way to eat broccoli is raw. But how do we do that without it feeling like some kind of raw foodist's self-punishment? After much trialling, I found that raw broccoli actually has a lovely sweet flavour – it's just the rock-hard texture that makes it tough going. When shredded finely to make a pesto, however, it is amazing tossed through hot pasta, stuffed into sandwiches, stirred through soups or scattered over a salad.

MAKES ABOUT 300G

PREP TIME 10 MINUTES

. . . .

1 HEAD OF BROCCOLI, ABOUT 300G,
CUT INTO FLORETS

80G PARMESAN CHEESE, GRATED

100G TOASTED FLAKED ALMONDS,
CHOPPED FINELY

FINELY GRATED ZEST AND JUICE OF 1 LEMON

100ML OLIVE OIL

1 TSP SALT

½ TSP BLACK PEPPER

SHRED the broccoli as finely as you can using a large knife. Much of the broccoli will crumble away, but the rest will form thin sheets, creating a lovely chunky texture.

PUT the shredded broccoli into a large bowl, add all the remaining ingredients and toss until well combined.

USE immediately or store the pesto in the fridge for up to 1 week.

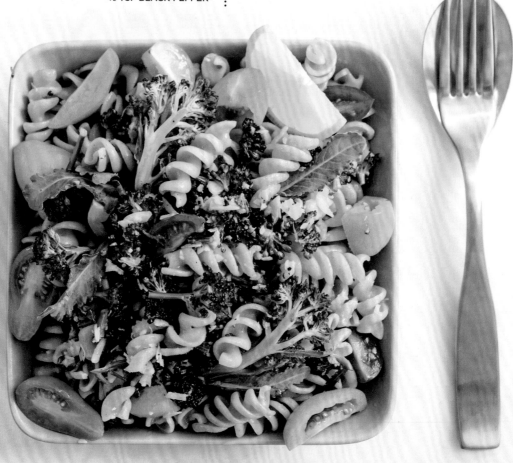

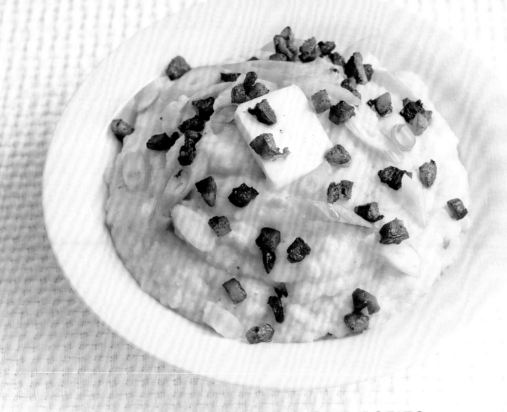

CAULIFLOWER MASHED POTATO

Mixing cauliflower into this mash reduces the total calories by a quarter, while sneaking in a whole extra serving of veg per person. This lazy one-pot method means nutrients aren't lost in the cooking water and, of course, one less pan is used in prep. Less washing up, fewer calories, more flavour and nutrition? Not a bad deal, really.

SERVES 4

PREP TIME 15 MINUTES

COOK TIME ABOUT 30 MINUTES

400G WAXY POTATOES
(THEY ARE HEALTHIER THAN FLOURY ONES),
UNPEELED AND FINELY DICED

400G CAULIFLOWER, FINELY DICED

500ML MILK

500ML WATER

100G SPRING ONIONS, FINELY SLICED

1 GARLIC CLOVE, MINCED

SALT AND PEPPER

TO SERVE

1 TBSP COOKED BACON BITS

1 TSP BUTTER

PLACE the potatoes, cauliflower, milk and measured water in a saucepan, bring to the boil and cook for 30 minutes until tender. Take the pan off the heat. (Do not strain the cooking liquid).

ADD the spring onions and garlic and mash the whole lot together until smooth. Season well with salt and pepper.

SPOON into a serving dish, scatter over the bacon and serve topped with the butter.

ONE-POT MAC & CHEESE

I know I risk messing with this comfort-food classic at my peril. But I promise you, this veg-enriched retake hasn't lost one bit of creamy, cheesy goodness, despite containing a whopping three times more veg than it does pasta. Made all in one pot (yes, this really does work), this simple cheat reduces fuss, mess and cooking time, while improving its silky texture and nutrient retention. Don't believe me? Try it out for yourself!

SERVES 2
PREP TIME 15 MINUTES
COOK TIME 20 MINUTES

....

200G WHOLEWHEAT PENNE OR MACARONI PASTA

1 LITRE MILK

200G WINTER SQUASH, GRATED

200G CAULIFLOWER, (ORANGE IF POSSIBLE), BROKEN INTO SMALL FLORETS, PLUS A COUPLE OF THE LEAVES, CHOPPED

200G LEEKS, TRIMMED, CLEANED AND FINELY SLICED

1 TSP GROUND NUTMEG

1 TSP PEPPER

½ TSP SALT

1 CHICKEN OR VEGETABLE STOCK CUBE, CRUMBLED

1 BAY LEAF

4 GARLIC CLOVES, MINCED

150G EXTRA MATURE CHEDDAR CHEESE, GRATED

75G PARMESAN CHEESE, GRATED

COMBINE all the ingredients except the garlic and cheeses in a large, shallow saucepan. Bring to the boil, then reduce the heat and simmer for 15 minutes until the pasta is tender.

STIR through the garlic and grated cheeses. Cover with a lid, take off the heat and leave to stand for 5 minutes to thicken.

VARIATIONS

PEA & ROCKET

Make the Mac & Cheese as above, stirring through 100g **frozen peas** and a large handful of **rocket** with the garlic and cheeses.

WILD MUSHROOM

Make the Mac & Cheese as above, adding 100g sautéed mixed **wild mushrooms** and 1 tsp **truffle oil** with the garlic and cheeses.

ASPARAGUS & CHERRY TOMATO

Make the Mac & Cheese as above, adding 100g blanched **asparagus spears** and 10–12 **cherry tomatoes** with the garlic and cheeses.

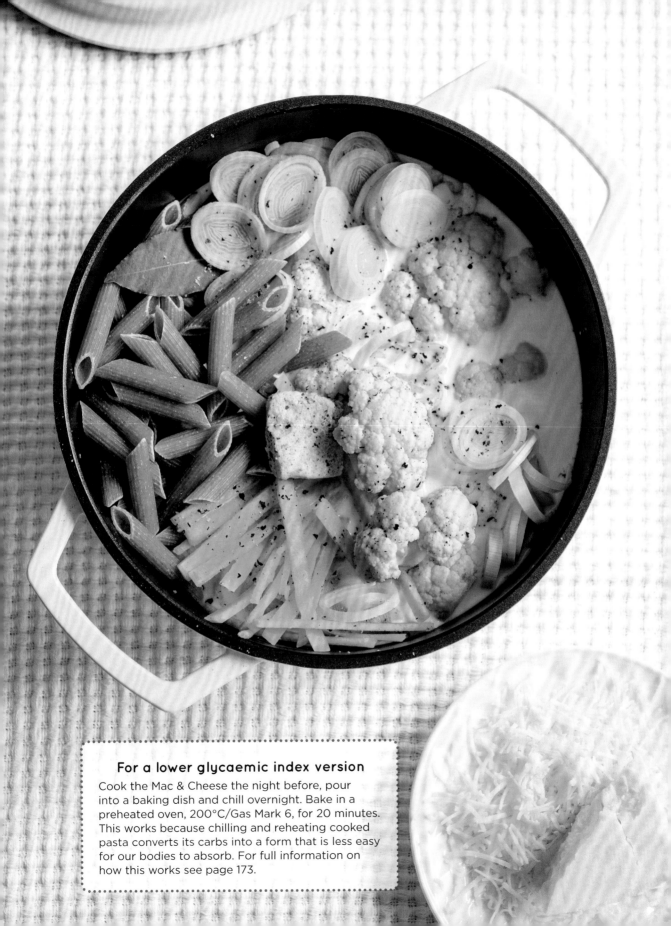

For a lower glycaemic index version

Cook the Mac & Cheese the night before, pour
into a baking dish and chill overnight. Bake in a
preheated oven, 200°C/Gas Mark 6, for 20 minutes.
This works because chilling and reheating cooked
pasta converts its carbs into a form that is less easy
for our bodies to absorb. For full information on
how this works see page 173.

POTATOES

Spuds have not had it easy lately. Amid the frenzied popularity of high-protein, low-carb diet regimes like Atkins and Paleo, they have often been demonized as a sort of dietary kryptonite – the source of quick, cheap energy that will pile on the pounds and even send your risk of diabetes shooting skywards. But, as always, the scientific evidence tells quite another story...

Rich in fibre, vitamin C and potassium, a range of studies has not only failed to find a consistent link between potato consumption and weight gain, but actually shows they can reduce blood pressure, decrease cholesterol and help calm inflammation. And with a few simple tips and tricks you can reap all these benefits without impacting your waistline. Here is my guide to curbing their carbs, while giving them a nutritional boost. Spud lovers, unite!

♡ SPUDS & HEALTHY WEIGHT

What makes this spud phobia particularly perplexing is that they actually contain far *fewer* calories gram for gram than almost all other starch sources, making them a low energy-density food roughly on a par with super-healthy beans – we are talking 50 per cent fewer calories than pasta and a whopping 70 per cent fewer than white bread.

Evidence shows that they are also better at inducing satiety – keeping you fuller for longer – according to a long-standing trial at the University of Sydney. Compared to white bread, rice and pasta, the team of Aussies found boiled potatoes stave off the physiological and psychological experiences of hunger more than two and a half times as long.

In fact, according to what appears to be the only clinical trial ever conducted to specifically look at the effects of potato consumption on body mass, published in the *Journal of Agricultural and Food Chemistry*, adding up to a hefty 16 (small) potatoes a day to participants' diets still resulted in zero weight gain. The extra potatoes appeared to keep the subjects so full, they just ate less of other things, and that can't be too bad a thing considering all the good stuff potatoes contain.

⚆ FULLER FOR LONGER?

Let's start with GI shall we? Short for 'Glycaemic Index', this stat refers to how quickly a food is digested and its energy released into your bloodstream in the form of sugar. The GI values for all foods are measured against a maximum score of 100, which is a dubious honour held by pure glucose and the almost instant sugar rush it gives you. The lower the score, the slower this energy is released and, generally speaking, the longer you feel full for. It's not an exact science, but a useful rough guide. As the GI for spuds varies widely between varieties, according to the *British Journal of Nutrition*, this could make the calories of some go a whole lot further than others.

PICK THE LITTLE GUYS

Up to 50 per cent of the polyphenols in potatoes come from their fibre-rich skin. The smaller the spud, the more skin they have, which means that by simply picking new potatoes over giant types you will get more phytonutrients. The indigestible fibre in the skin also slows the absorption of the carbohydrate, lowering their GI. From a lazy cook's point of view, their small size and thin skins mean they also require far less scrubbing and slicing, and of course no peeling. Being cooked whole also means they tend to lose less of their phytonutrients to the cooking water.

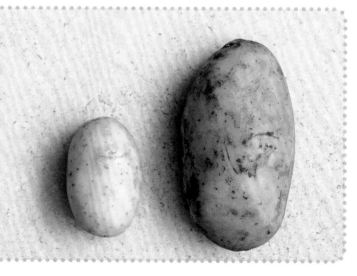

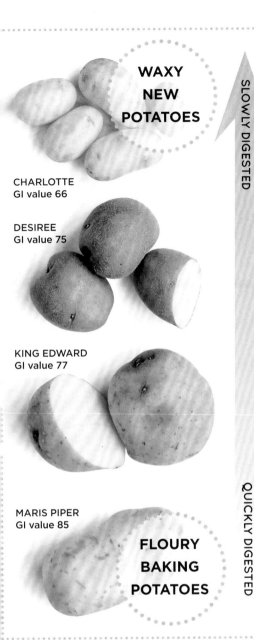

WAXY NEW POTATOES

CHARLOTTE
GI value 66

DESIREE
GI value 75

KING EDWARD
GI value 77

MARIS PIPER
GI value 85

FLOURY BAKING POTATOES

SLOWLY DIGESTED

QUICKLY DIGESTED

Charlotte & Nicola

New potatoes like Charlotte and Nicola tend to have the highest amount of a slowly digested, waxy-textured carb called amylose, giving them not only a deliciously slippery, moreish texture, but also the lowest spike in blood sugar. So much so that these two varieties are considered medium GI foods, putting them alongside foods like wholegrain bread and bananas. Nicola, in particular, has a GI value so low it's a borderline low GI food. And if that wasn't enough, their firm consistency also causes them to hold their shape better when cooked and mop up less grease than any other type.

Desiree & King Edward

These typical middle-of-the-road potatoes don't fill you up for as long and tend to be slightly fluffier in texture than the waxy types. This is because they contain less satisfying amylose and more of a different type of carb called amylopectin. This has a floury, powdery texture and is far easier for our bodies to digest, giving you a much faster rise in blood sugar than baby and new potatoes, but this is nothing compared to the almost instant sugar rush of baking/mashing types.

Maris Piper

With a sky-high GI value (much higher than the average potato), large, floury spuds like Maris Piper are typically used to bake or mash. They contain loads of mealy, easy-to-digest amylopectin and the lowest quantity of filling amylose, which gives you a very quick energy hit, but as a consequence might leave you peckish pretty soon after. Their porous, light-as-a-cloud consistency sadly means they tend to require a larger amount of butter or oil to compensate for a 'powdery' mouthfeel, which they soak up like a sponge, so dishes made with them can contain higher fat levels, too.

SLICE, THEN ICE

When you buy potatoes in the shops they often have been stored for many months, sometimes up to 1 year. Sounds terrible, right? Well, according to a plethora of studies, the phytonutrients in harvested potatoes not only remain stable, but can even actually increase dramatically over time. In the refrigerated conditions of commercial storage, the still-living spuds start churning out these protective compounds to defend themselves against the chilly temperatures. And the great news is, according to researchers at Texas A&M University, you can speed this up at home by subjecting your spuds to just a little more stress. By simply slicing them into 5mm-thick pieces and bunging them in the fridge, this combination of mechanical damage to the cells and the cold can trigger them into almost doubling their antioxidants in just 2 days. OK, so this does require quite a lot of forward planning, but is easy to do if you have the time, and comes with a pretty big potential benefit.

PURPLE PROMISE

Want to go one better? Pick a fancy burgundy-fleshed variety of potato, like Purple Majesty or Violetta, and you get not only hypnotic colour, but also up to four times the antioxidant activity. Packed full of the same pigments that give red wine and blueberries their potential health benefits, these spuds boast three times the polyphenols of the regular kind. In fact, gram for gram they can contain just as much of the good stuff as berries themselves, according to Colorado State University, and yet cost 90 per cent less at my local supermarket. Trust me, I'm a geek, I did the maths.

But what does all this actually mean in terms of your health? Well, for starters, one trial published in the *Journal of Agricultural and Food Chemistry* found that adding a 140g serving of purple potatoes twice a day to the diet of overweight, middle-aged subjects caused their blood pressure to drop almost 5 points within just a month – despite the fact that almost 80 per cent of them were already on antihypotensive drugs. Such a fall could, statistically speaking, 'decrease the risk of stroke by over 30 per cent and of heart disease by 20 per cent and reduce the likelihood of dementia, heart failure, and mortality from cardiovascular disease', according to the Royal London School of Medicine. And even though these potatoes added a sizeable 280 calories to their daily diet, the subjects didn't gain weight.

But that's not the end of the story. Other human trials have found that consuming purple potatoes, even in half the doses of the above, could reduce DNA damage and inflammation associated with chronic disease and have far less impact on blood sugar than regular spuds.

Of course, potato plants don't produce this dazzling purple colour for our benefit. One theory is that the antimicrobial properties of anthocyanins help protect the plant from a debilitating fungal infection called blight, which strikes worst in cool, wet conditions. In fact, a number of trials have shown that purple spuds grown in cooler climates with longer summer days and higher rainfall (such as that of the UK) tend to churn out as much as two and a half times more anthocyanins and loads more antioxidants. This means for me, as a Londoner at least, buying local could be a measurably healthier choice. Well, why not?

THE GOODNESS IS SKIN DEEP

The skin of spuds contains more than double the total polyphenols of the flesh itself and a huge proportion of their essential vitamins and minerals. This means that simply not bothering to peel them could prevent the loss of roughly half the iron, along with a third of the calcium and, in purple varieties, almost half the heart-healthy anthocyanin pigments that you'd otherwise just be chucking in the bin. Boiling potatoes whole in their skins also prevents loss of nutrients that would otherwise leach into the cooking water through the cut surfaces. Coming pre-wrapped in an edible, nutrient-rich package that seals goodness in, I don't know why anyone would waste their time peeling. You can always slice them after cooking if you want, but most people will barely notice a difference in taste or texture if you leave the peel on.

MICROWAVE OR BOIL

There have been loads of studies over the years that have investigated the effect of different cooking methods. Although the results have varied, there does seem to be an emerging pattern, which a comprehensive new study published in the journal *Food Chemistry* nicely reflects. More than any other method, of eight different cooking methods tested, microwaving whole potatoes in the skin consistently proved the best at retaining pretty much every nutrient, closely followed by boiling them whole in their skins. Steaming and baking were roughly on a par, but a definitive step down from the previous two methods. Worst of all was frying, but I bet you already guessed that.

Violetta

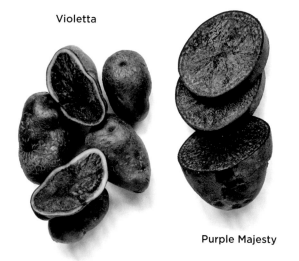

Purple Majesty

PURPLE POTATO SALAD WITH FETA, PEAS, POMEGRANATE & HERBS

There is one simple trick that can slash the calories in potatoes while simultaneously quelling their impact on blood sugar by as much as 37 per cent, turning spuds from a high GI food to one or two points away from being classified as low. All you have to do is cook them the night before and chill them for 24 hours in the fridge. This period of cold causes some of their starch molecules to expand and crystallize – a chemical change that turns them into what is known as 'resistant starch' (see page 106). Even if reheated, this starch can no longer be digested by the human body, effectively transforming it, almost as if by magic, from calorie-rich carb to healthy fibre.

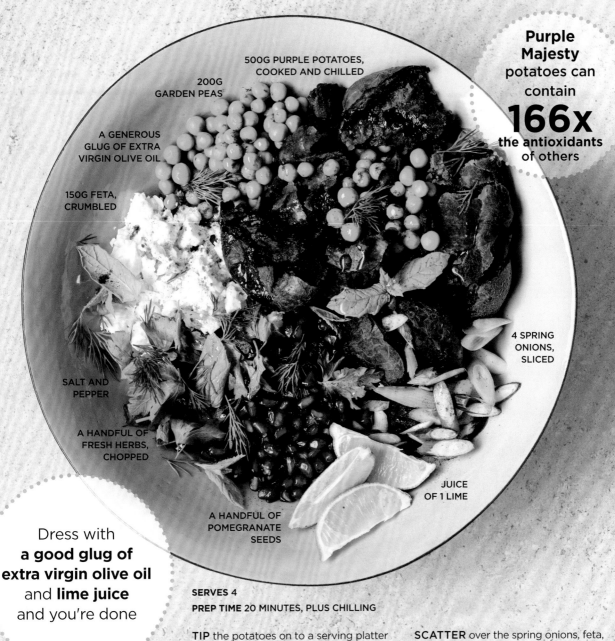

500G PURPLE POTATOES, COOKED AND CHILLED

200G GARDEN PEAS

A GENEROUS GLUG OF EXTRA VIRGIN OLIVE OIL

150G FETA, CRUMBLED

SALT AND PEPPER

A HANDFUL OF FRESH HERBS, CHOPPED

A HANDFUL OF POMEGRANATE SEEDS

JUICE OF 1 LIME

4 SPRING ONIONS, SLICED

Purple Majesty potatoes can contain

166x

the antioxidants of others

Dress with **a good glug of extra virgin olive oil** and **lime juice** and you're done

SERVES 4
PREP TIME 20 MINUTES, PLUS CHILLING

TIP the potatoes on to a serving platter and crush them roughly with the back of a fork.

SCATTER over the spring onions, feta, peas, pomegranate seeds and herbs. Drizzle over the olive oil and lime juice and season to taste.

SWEET POTATOES

With twice the fibre and one and a half times the vitamin C of the humble spud, sweet potatoes pack a pretty hefty punch in the nutritional stakes. An extremely rich source of antioxidant carotenes, just one small serving of sweet potato offers up all the vitamin A you need in a day and more (higher than any other root vegetable), plus significantly more potassium, calcium and vitamin K, all for roughly the same calories as regular potatoes.

They even have a much lower GI (see page 46) than spuds, so you will be kept fuller for longer, too, despite their far more sugary flavour. All in all, a pretty sweet deal, really. In a health-food face-off, I know which one my money would be on.

VARIETY IS KEY

The nutritional differences between sweet potato cultivars are probably the greatest of any crop in this book. Picking one over another could give you (a frankly, insane) 316 times the polyphenols for the same amount of calories. Fortunately, a team at North Carolina State University (ground zero for sweet potato cultivation and research) have tested 19 different varieties to create a handy league table for you, ranking them by their polyphenol content.

Purple sweet potatoes contain 3X the antioxidants of blueberries

Stokes Purple

Purple varieties are given their dazzling colour by the same antioxidant pigments (called anthocyanins) that are believed to give blueberries their health benefits. In fact, gram for gram they contain three times as many as the celebrated 'superfruit'. With more than four and a half times the antioxidants of its closest nutritional rival Evangeline, Stokes Purple is one of the most nutritious of all the purple varieties according to the North Carolinians and also happens to be the easiest to track down in fancier supermarkets. Purple varieties also have the lowest GI of all sweet potatoes, which could help keep hunger pangs at bay. They even have denser, less watery flesh and a richer flavour than the orange ones too. A pretty perfect combination all round it seems.

Evangeline

When it comes to the more commonly sold orange sweet potato cultivars, the same team from North Carolina State revealed that Evangeline came out head and shoulders above the rest in terms of carotene content, boasting 60 per cent more than the supermarket staple Covington. This richness of carotenes gives Evangeline its deep orange hue, added antioxidant activity and vitamin A content. If that wasn't enough, because the aroma chemicals that give sweet potato its characteristic nutty, buttery flavour are generated by a breakdown of carotenes, Evangeline is queen of the culinary stakes, too.

Covington

Most sweet potatoes in supermarkets don't come with variety labels. That's because one variety called Covington is so dominant on the shelves that until very recently there weren't really any other options. If it doesn't have a label, this will be it. Although Covington isn't quite as high in carotenes as Evangeline, it does come a close second, being higher than any of the other varieties tested, according to the North Carolinians.

O'Henry

It's hard not to be mean about the cream-fleshed varieties. Aside from the fact that they can contain 90 per cent less antioxidant activity than the purple types (on average), and just a tiny fraction of the polyphenols, they also have a higher GI, which means you could be eyeing up the snacks come mid-afternoon. In certain areas of Africa where white sweet potatoes are a staple crop, research has shown that simply swapping to orange varieties could help eliminate the widespread vitamin A deficiencies that affect up to 68 per cent of all children. Did I mention orange ones are sweeter and more aromatic, too?

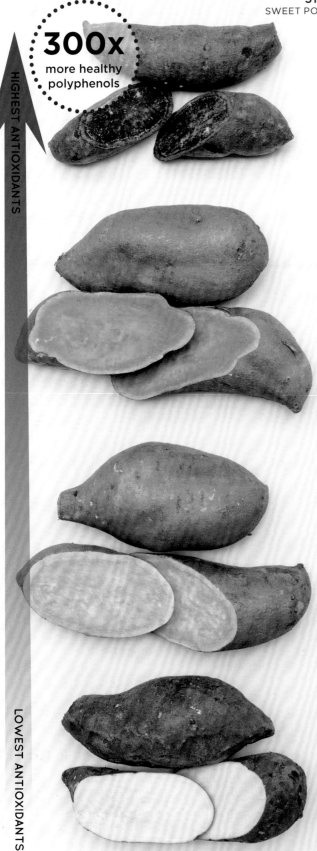

HIGHEST ANTIOXIDANTS

300x
more healthy polyphenols

LOWEST ANTIOXIDANTS

POWER OF PURPLE

With their hefty dose of anthocyanins, purple sweet potatoes, in particular, have attracted the attention of researchers, with a few emerging studies unearthing some intriguing results.

Lowering of blood pressure

In animal studies consuming purple sweet potatoes has been found to help significantly lower cholesterol. But could it do the same in humans? A small 2014 clinical trial reported in the *Journal of Biology, Agriculture and Healthcare* aimed to find out. The Indonesian researchers discovered that after just a month of consuming a daily 180ml dose of a drink made from purple sweet potatoes, elderly patients with hypertension saw significant falls in their blood pressure, enough to take them from advanced stage 2 hypertension to borderline prehypertension. That's about the equivalent of a modest half a serving per day to potentially lower your statistical risk of heart disease. Medicine never tasted so good.

Liver protection

Another small trial, this time in Japan, found that a similar dose of a purple sweet potato drink could reduce the markers of liver damage in men with borderline hepatitis, suggesting that the beneficial effect of sweet potatoes could have a protective effect not just against the risk of heart disease, but other areas of the body too.

Brain boost

A number of animal trials have suggested that extracts of purple sweet potato could help protect brain cells against damage from toxins that mimic the effect of ageing. Rats fed with these extracts were able to navigate mazes far more quickly, demonstrating enhanced memory and spatial learning. The researchers even reported a reversal in the damage in rats that consumed the purple sweet potato products, concluding that 'the age-related impairment in learning and memory may be relieved by antioxidant treatment'. Well, at least in rats.

THE DARKER THE BETTER

Even between purple varieties, there can be a wide variation in the levels of anthocyanins they contain. With darker Stokes Purple boasting up to five times the anthocyanins of the lighter, lavender-hued Okinawan, pick the darkest every time.

BAKE FOR THE MOST NUTRIENTS

According to a study published in the journal *Food and Nutrition Sciences*, while boiling or microwaving boosted sweet potatoes' heart-healthy polyphenols by an impressive 50 per cent, baking them worked even better, causing a threefold increase. And the benefits don't end there. In the case of the purple varieties, their heart-healthy anthocyanins can be degraded as much as 20 per cent by steaming, microwaving, frying or pressure-cooking, according to Kansas State University. Baking them, however, kept 100 per cent of these purple pigments intact, helping preserve their potential health benefits and vivid colour.

Even in the orange varieties, baking shows a positive effect, giving your veg 30 per cent more vitamin A over boiled, according to the United States Department of Agriculture (USDA). This works because baking them also helps reduce the water content of the roots, concentrating their sugary flavour and preventing key nutrients and flavour from leaching into cooking water. Baking is also by far the easiest cooking method: no chopping, no peeling, no draining, just wrap the sweet potatoes in foil and bung them in the oven at 160°C for 1–1½ hours, depending on the size of your spuds. This may be a good 40°C lower than some recipes recommend, but it will help the sweet potatoes retain significantly more of the colour, particularly in purple varieties, that can be destroyed at higher temperatures. After countless kitchen experiments, I have found that the foil wrapping, despite not making the sweet potatoes cook any faster, does result in a softer, easier-to-eat skin. Much more pleasant than the leathery effect you get by baking them unwrapped. The foil jacket also appears to help retain a much better colour, keeping more of those all-important phytonutrients intact.

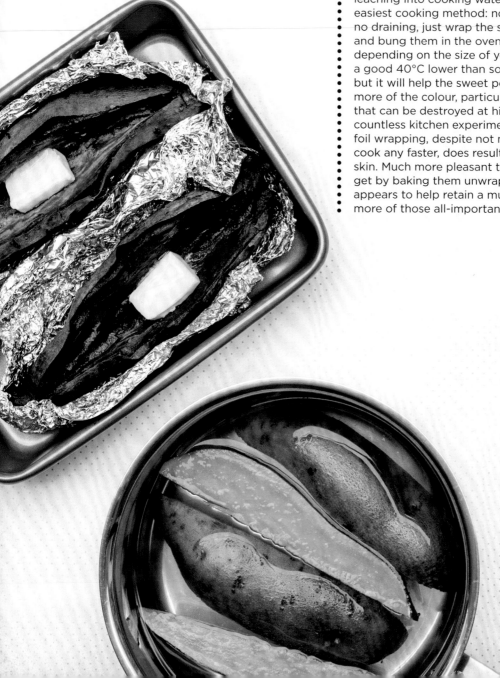

BE LAZY & INDULGE

Want to get even more of the good stuff? Here are three more simple tips on how to do just that by doing less work and getting more flavour:

Don't bother peeling

Antioxidant activity in sweet potato skin can be up to four times higher than the flesh itself, according to USDA. Simply don't bother peeling them, for loads more fibre and higher polyphenols too.

Love leftovers

As with potatoes (see page 49), precooking and cooling sweet potatoes can up their content of resistant starch by 62 per cent, according to the *International Journal of Food Science and Nutrition*, keeping you fuller for longer, slashing calories and boosting your friendly gut bacteria. But who has the time? Precooking can actually mean *less* effort too. Next time you are baking a batch of sweet potatoes, just do twice the amount. The wrapped leftovers will last for up to a week in the fridge in a plastic container, giving you a supply of lower GI carbs that can be heated up in the microwave in 2 minutes flat.

Don't skip the fat

Adding a drizzle of extra virgin olive oil at serving time can help your body absorb significantly more of the betacarotene. This is a great idea even for purple varieties, as many of these can contain significant amounts of this orange pigment albeit disguised by the bright purple anthocyanins. This extra fat can also help slow the digestion of carbs, effectively lowering the GI and thereby keeping you satiated.

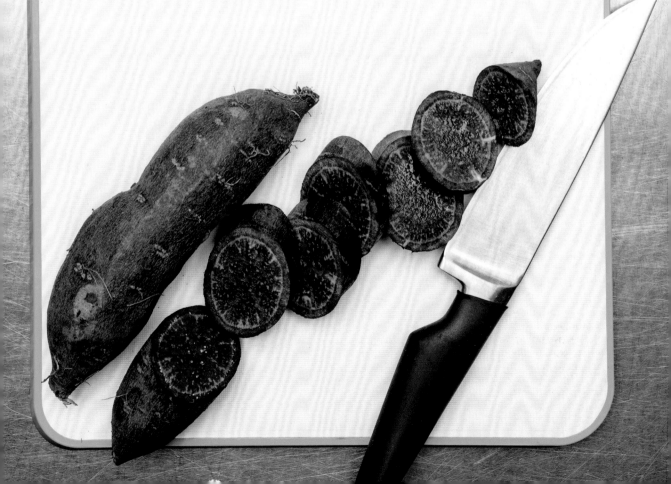

DOUBLE SWEET POTATO PIE

Sticky sweet, an amazing colour and made with over 50 per cent fruit, veg and nuts, this is my nutrient-dense, no-added-sugar take on the soul-food classic. I am way too lazy to spend hours rolling out pastry, so I have concocted a super-easy crust using little more than sweet potatoes, coconut and almonds that takes 5 minutes to make.

SERVES 6

PREP TIME 25 MINUTES, PLUS COOLING

COOK TIME 1 HOUR 20 MINUTES

CRUST

100G ORANGE SWEET POTATO, GRATED

100G GROUND ALMONDS

50G DESICCATED COCONUT

2 EGG WHITES

1 TBSP GRANULATED STEVIA (BAKING BLEND)

FILLING

2 EGGS

100G GRANULATED STEVIA (BAKING BLEND)

½ TSP SALT

½ TSP GROUND NUTMEG

1 TSP CINNAMON

500G COOKED PURPLE SWEET POTATO

TO DECORATE

BLACKBERRIES

MINT LEAVES

SHREDDED COCONUT

PREHEAT the oven to 200°C/Gas Mark 6, and line a 25cm flan tin with baking paper.

FIRST, make the crust. Squeeze the grated sweet potato over the sink to extract as much liquid as possible, then transfer to a bowl and combine with the remaining crust ingredients to form a dough. Press the mixture firmly into the base and sides of the prepared tin.

BAKE for 15–20 minutes, or until golden. Use a spoon to further compact the crust into the sides and base of the tin, then leave to cool slightly. Reduce the oven temperature to 150°C/Gas Mark 2.

MEANWHILE, make the filling. Blitz all the ingredients together in a food processor until you have a smooth, velvety mixture.

POUR the filling over the crust and bake for 1 hour, or until the filling is set with a very slight wobble in the centre. Leave the pie to cool completely.

DECORATE the pie with blackberries, mint leaves and grated coconut.

SWEET STEVIA

I have a notoriously sweet tooth, but I have found that granulated stevia (made using the zero-calorie, naturally-sweet compounds found in stevia plants) is a virtually indistinguishable substitute for sugar in recipes like this. There are several types available. For the recipes in this book I use 'baking blends' formulated to be of equal sweetness to sugar. Check the label as some versions are far sweeter than sugar spoon for spoon.

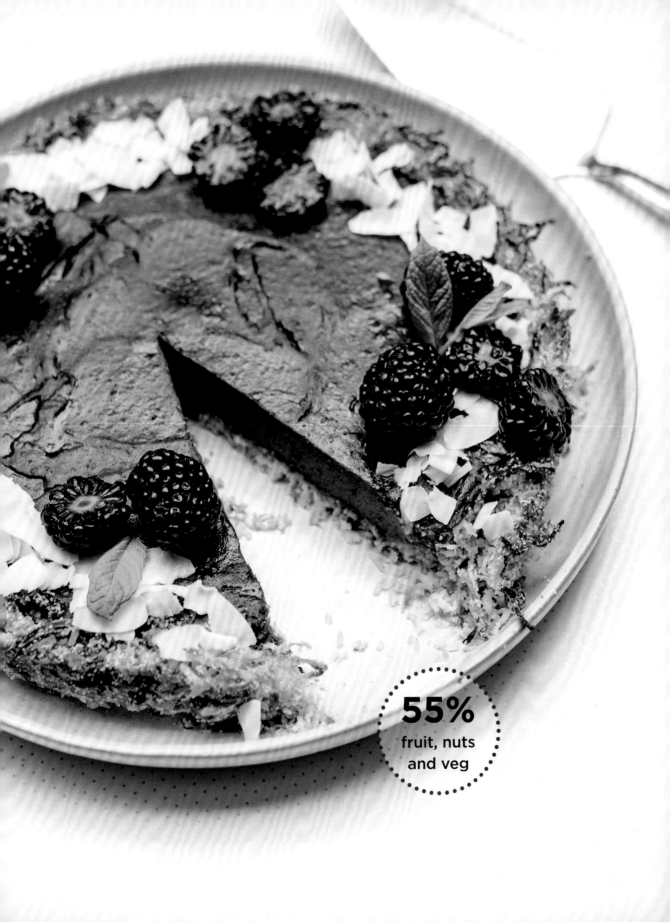

55%
fruit, nuts
and veg

SWEET POTATO & PECAN DOUGHNUTS

They look like doughnuts, taste like carrot cake and, shockingly, are made up of about 70 per cent fruit, nuts and veg. In fact there's so much good stuff in here that there's almost no room left for added sugar or fat. One of my all-time favourite recipes, I went through 14 different versions before I finally got these spot on.

MAKES 9 DOUGHNUTS
PREP TIME 20 MINUTES, PLUS COOLING
COOK TIME 30 MINUTES

OLIVE OIL, FOR GREASING
120G WHOLEMEAL FLOUR
1 TSP BAKING POWDER
1 TSP MIXED SPICE
½ TSP SALT
3 TBSP GRANULATED STEVIA (BAKING BLEND) OR SOFT BROWN SUGAR
1 TSP VANILLA EXTRACT
1 EGG
1 SMALL BANANA
350G COOKED ORANGE SWEET POTATO
50G PECAN NUTS, CHOPPED

TO DECORATE
MELTED CHOCOLATE (DARK OR WHITE)
CHOPPED DRIED FRUIT (I USED GOJI BERRIES AND FREEZE-DRIED STRAWBERRIES)
CHOPPED NUTS (I USED FLAKED ALMONDS AND DESICCATED COCONUT)

PREHEAT the oven to 180°C/Gas Mark 4. Grease 9 sections of an 8.5cm doughnut tray lightly with a little oil.

WHISK the flour, baking powder, mixed spice, salt and stevia or sugar together in a large mixing bowl.

BLITZ the vanilla extract, egg, banana and sweet potato together in a food processor until smooth, then fold into the flour mixture with the pecans.

SPOON the mixture into the prepared doughnut sections and bake for 30 minutes, or until risen and golden. Leave to cool.

DECORATE the doughnuts with melted chocolate, dried fruit and chopped nuts. I added a couple of drops of natural pink food colouring to some white chocolate to give these doughnuts added prettiness, but plain dark or white chocolate work just as well.

DOUGHNUTS THAT ARE OUT OF THIS WORLD

Sweet potatoes are so high in key nutrients that they have been extensively tested at the Kennedy Space Center as part of the rations of NASA astronauts, according to a 1998 study. Reading through scientific reports on how they were turned into pancakes, waffles, tortillas, bread, pie, pound cake, pasta, doughnuts and pretzels, I thought 'I could do that!' So this is my NASA-inspired doughnut recipe with over three times the sweet potato than even the space program could cram in.

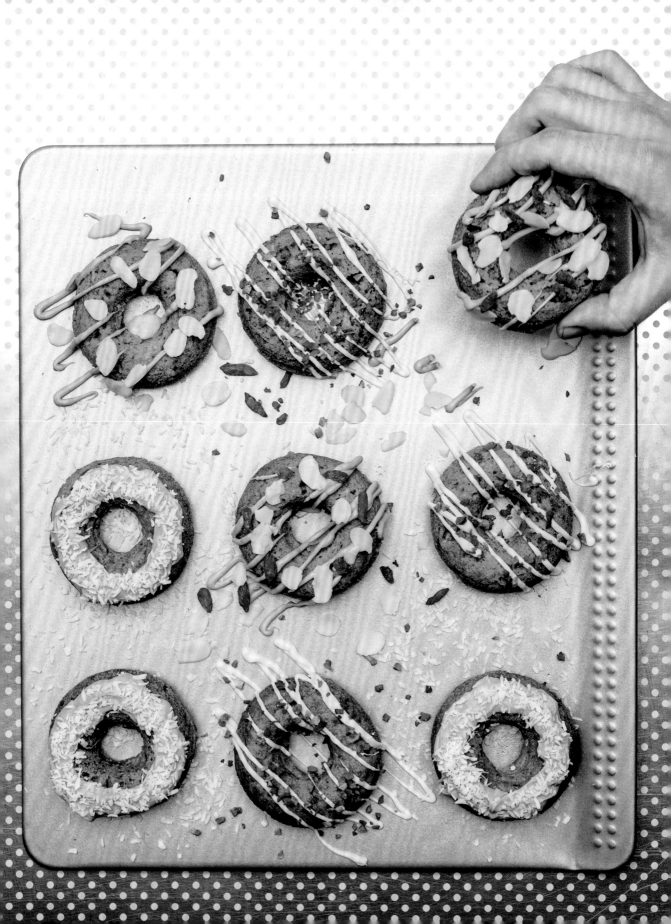

ONIONS & GARLIC

Probably the two most commonly used medicinal plants on the planet, onions and garlic contain a range of antioxidant and anti-inflammatory compounds that a growing stack of clinical trials suggests may be useful in preventing a host of degenerative diseases. Yet as the levels of the beneficial chemicals can differ enormously between varieties and even according to how they are prepared and eaten, in fact by up to a hundredfold, a little knowledge could make a huge difference to their nutrition. And that is what this section is all about...

♡ BLOOD THINNERS?

When you slice into an onion or garlic bulb you spark off chemical reactions that churn out pungent sulphur-based compounds at the site of the wound, which are designed to protect the plant from infection. It's these antioxidant chemicals that give both these veg their characteristic spicy flavour when raw and part of their potential health benefits. Along with polyphenols like quercetin that onions are also rich in, these compounds have been demonstrated by a growing body of research to act as natural blood thinners, preventing cell fragments called platelets from clumping together to form clots. This is intriguing as increasing amounts of these platelet clusters are associated with a much higher risk of heart attack and stroke. As garlic produces far more of these sulphurous chemicals, its blood-thinning powers are 13 times greater gram for gram than onions, according to Denmark's University of Odense. Ever noticed that raw garlic is way more pungent tasting than the same quantity of raw onion? That's why.

♡ BUSTING HYPERTENSION

A comprehensive review of the best available clinical trials from all over the world by the University of Adelaide found that garlic significantly beat placebo pills at lowering blood pressure in people with hypertension, with an average reduction of 7 points in diastolic blood pressure. These are some fascinating findings because a decrease of just 5 points is associated with over a 20 per cent reduction in the risk of experiencing a heart attack and heart failure along with a 40 per cent lower risk of stroke, a reduction similar to that found in some prescription drugs! While there is currently not enough evidence to suggest those on blood pressure meds should be tempted to switch to garlic (crucially, none of these trials actually directly compared its effects against conventional drugs), adding a little more of this tasty veg to your diet might well be a good idea. Watch this space for more info.

♡ LOWERING CHOLESTEROL

The same team of Adelaide data geeks didn't stop at blood pressure. In a second study, they trawled through the findings from 39 trials that tested the effect of garlic preparations on cardiovascular health and discovered that on average subjects with high cholesterol saw their levels drop by 8 per cent after consuming garlic for 2 months, all with little or no side effects. While this may not sound like very much, a reduction of this scale is statistically associated with about a 40 per cent reduction in risk of coronary events at 50 years of age, leading the researchers to go as far as concluding that garlic 'might be considered as an alternative option with a higher safety profile than conventional cholesterol-lowering medications in patients with slightly elevated cholesterol'. OK, that's a pretty big 'might', but nevertheless some amazing results for an ingredient in everyone's kitchen cupboard.

♡ GUT HEALTH

On top of loads of healthy polyphenols and sulphur-based compounds, both garlic and onions contain large amounts of indigestible carbohydrates called oligosaccharides, which act like fibre in our digestive tract. While we can't access the energy they contain, the friendly bacteria that live in our gut positively thrive on the stuff. This is good news as there is an increasing weight of solid science to suggest that healthy populations of these microbes can significantly reduce your risk of bowel cancer, improve your immune function and even potentially reduce feelings of depression and anxiety. In fact, on a serving-by-serving basis, onions appear to be one of the top three dietary sources (alongside artichokes and leeks) among everyday fruit and veg to feed the little guys with.

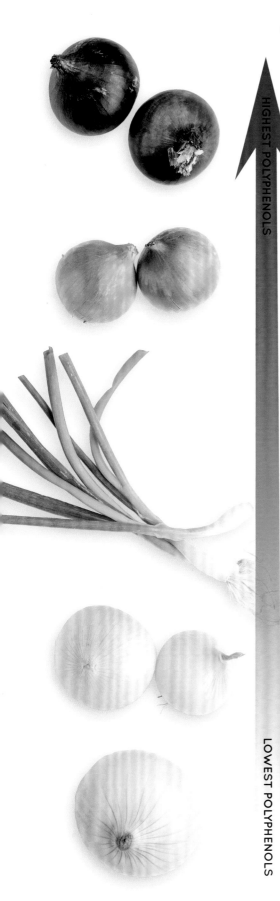

HIGHEST POLYPHENOLS

LOWEST POLYPHENOLS

Red & brown onions

Containing up to one hundred times the polyphenols of white varieties, both brown and red onions are hands down much better sources of these key antioxidants than their paler cousins. But a range of studies suggests that red seems to have the edge. The exact amount does appear to vary according to which varieties you choose to include in your comparisons (there are hundreds out there), with different studies showing different values. However, red varieties with an extra 60–70 per cent more polyphenols than brown are not unusual. This phenomenon might well be owing to the antioxidant anthocyanin pigments (a key group of polyphenols) that give the red kind their pretty coloration. Go for the strongest-flavoured, most pungent types to get the heftiest dose of the healthy sulphur-based chems too.

Spring onions

Spring onions are not simply younger versions of regular onions like their name suggests. In fact, they actually belong to an entirely different species (*Allium fistulosum*), sometimes called green onions or Welsh onions. Japanese researchers looked into their phytonutrient value and found that both the polyphenol content and total antioxidant content were just slightly lower than those of brown onions, yet significantly higher than white varieties.

White onions

White onions have been consistently shown to have the lowest levels of polyphenols, of all standard varieties, in trial after trial, with on average less than 1 per cent of the regular brown or red varieties, according to a study of 75 cultivars at Texas A&M University. In fact, in over half the white onion varieties tested, levels of blood pressure-lowering quercetin were so low they could not even be detected. As these are harder to track down and often sold at premium prices, I'd sidestep them every time.

Supersweet onions

When Cornell University researchers analysed the new 'supersweet' onions that are increasingly popular in the US and UK, they found that trendy new hybrids were even lower in polyphenols than standard white onions. And that's saying something. These onions are given their supersweet flavour not by a sky-high sugar content, but from extremely low levels of the beneficial sulphur-based chemicals – without much pungency, the sensation of sweetness comes to the fore. This may explain why the Cornell team also found that supersweets have half the cancer-fighting ability on tumour cells cultured in test tubes compared with standard onions. The very least pungent types have also been found to contain the lowest amounts of prebiotics. If it's phytonutrients you are after, give these guys a wide berth.

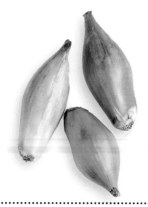

🧺 SUPER SHALLOTS

There is one onion relative out there that knocks the socks off even the very best conventional types, according to a growing number of studies: the shallot. With as much as six times more polyphenols than some everyday onions, these fancy French types outshone all of the top ten cultivars on sale in the USA in the antioxidant stakes in a trial published in the *Journal of Agricultural and Food Chemistry*. Even when going head-to-head with nutrient-rich red onions, shallots were shown to have more than three times the antioxidants by Washington State University.

🍲 COOKED OR RAW?

Is it better to cook garlic and onions or eat them raw? Well, the answer is 'both', according to the latest scientific research.

Raw is best for blood thinning

To a plant geek like me, the sulphur compounds believed to be primarily responsible for the anti-clotting effects of onions and garlic are truly fascinating. You see, these pungent defence chemicals, designed to kill bacteria, viruses and fungi, ironically also happen to be toxic to the very plant that makes them. For this reason they are only ever produced at the site of a wound, when ruptured cells burst open causing two chemicals – a benign precursor and an enzyme called alliinase – to mix (a bit like when you crack a glowstick; 90s kids, remember those?).

The tricky thing is that alliinase isn't heat stable, meaning that as soon as you cook onions or garlic you stop their ability to make anti-clotting agents dead in its tracks. For this reason, eating them raw is consistently reported to be the best bet for full blood-thinning benefit.

Cooked is best for polyphenols & prebiotics

Quercetin, the main polyphenol in onions, on the other hand, has been shown to be remarkably resistant to heat. In fact, its levels can actually be raised by cooking by as much as 50 per cent. This is thought to be because cooking breaks open the tissues in which it is stored, releasing the cholesterol-lowering quercetin and thus making it more easily absorbed.

While cooking onions can knock their levels of prebiotics back by as much as 40 per cent, according to the United States Department of Agriculture, it also softens the texture of veg, shrinking its volume and quelling its pungent bite. This means you can consume far more of them in a single serving, about four times more according to my own kitchen experiments.

🍲 THE BEST OF BOTH WORLDS

Fortunately, for those who aren't fans of the fiery bite of raw onions or garlic, food scientists have uncovered two ridiculously simple cheats that can, as if by magic, send the levels of sulphur compounds in cooked onions and garlic soaring, while retaining their superior quercetin content. Do either and see a potential spike in phytonutrient content; do both and of course you get even more.

Cut & run

First, while alliinase may be terribly susceptible to heat, the sulphur chemicals it produces (the stuff that actually does you good) are far more tolerant to cooking. According to a team of Argentinian researchers, that means if you simply slice your onions and garlic and leave them to rest for 10–20 minutes – enough time for the chemical reaction to take place – they will retain far more of their benefits even after cooking. But who has time to stop everything and wait around for 20 minutes in the kitchen? The wonderful news is, you don't have to. Simply tweak the order of cooking to chop the onions or garlic at the very start – then carry on with the rest of the prep. By the time you are ready so will be the newly nutritionally-charged veg.

Replace with raw

Perhaps the weirdest thing about these veg is that even once simmered to a point where all alliinase has been wiped out, there is still plenty of the precursor left in the cooked onions and garlic. As the raw veg boast super-concentrated doses of the all-important enzyme, according to the Argentinian team, adding tiny amounts of them to finished meals and waiting a few minutes before serving can trigger off the same chemical reaction. As little as 10 per cent of the amount of cooked garlic in a recipe added at the end of cooking in raw form can restore 100 per cent of its anti-clotting benefits. And, theoretically speaking, similar results should be found in onions, too.

USE OLD GARLIC

Old garlic bulbs, especially those that have started to sprout, have been shown to manufacture far more of the sulphur-based chemicals, sending their antioxidant content soaring, a phenomenon that is almost certainly due to the bulbs' attempts to defend themselves against stress. If fresh garlic is super-healthy, that old garlic you have knocking about at the back of your cupboard is likely to be even better and with a much stronger flavour to boot. Don't bin it, eat it.

DRIED GARLIC IS GREAT

You might think that processed garlic powder is a terrible cheat, with all its goodness obliterated by the drying and grinding that gives it its long shelf life and wonderful convenience. Yet nothing could be further from the truth. In fact, when you look at the stack of studies that report garlic's benefits, they have not been done using fresh cloves at all but on garlic extracts, in particular the dried powdered form. However, as the chemical reactions that generate the beneficial compounds are destroyed when they meet the acid of your stomach, many garlic pills are coated to prevent them from dissolving until they reach the neutral pH of the intestine. But there is a way around this!

Simply rehydrating dried garlic powder for 30 minutes at room temperature will activate the enzyme and give the reaction enough time to kick out the good stuff before hitting your stomach, according to Oregon State University. All you have to do is mix it with a tablespoon of water at the start of your recipes, then carry on as normal and add it to the pan at the end and you can save yourself the hassle of peeling and chopping. Alternatively, sprinkle it into dressings, sauces or over tomato salads and wait 30 minutes before serving for full benefit with zero work.

Garlic has

13x

the **blood-thinning powers** of **onions**

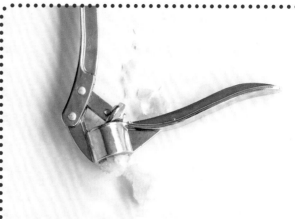

LOVE THE GARLIC PRESS

The finer you chop onions or garlic and the more damage you inflict, the more anti-clotting sulphur compounds that you'll generate. In the case of garlic, whacking whole cloves – skin and all – in a garlic press creates way more damage than laborious chopping by hand in exchange for much less effort. It's my all-time favourite kitchen tool.

TACKLING GARLIC BREATH

Here's the million-dollar question: can you really get the full benefits of garlic and still keep your friends? After all, it is the self-same sulphurous compounds linked to their heart-healthy properties that also cause their inevitable after-effects. While there might be all sorts of foods traditionally believed to mop up the dragon breath – from mint and parsley to green tea and spinach, and even plain old milk – which of these actually work? Well, apparently, all of them, according to two trials at the Ohio State University, reducing some of the sulphur compounds emitted in human breath by about 90 per cent. Of the three leafy greens tested, all had a broadly similar level of efficacy compared to the control, with mint having a slight edge on spinach and parsley. While milk could help freshen breath even hours after scoffing the garlic, consuming it together with veg had an even more pronounced effect, with creamy whole milk being measurably more effective than watery skimmed. Hooray for full-fat.

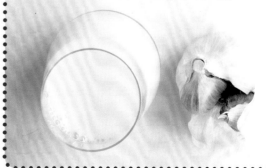

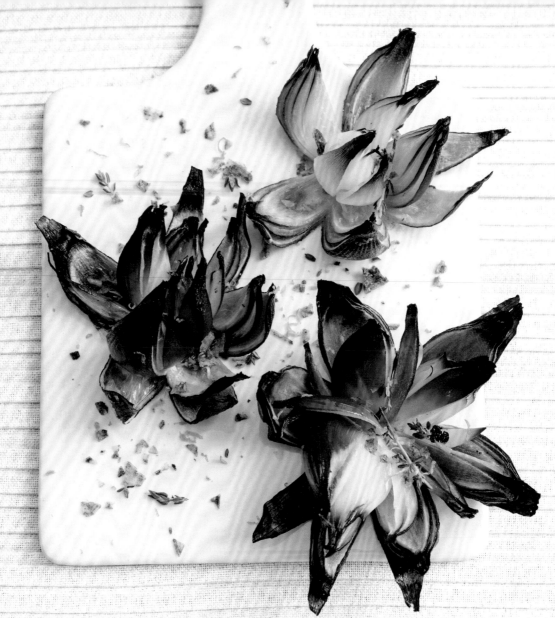

ROASTED ONION 'FLOWERS'

Onions seem to be forever a 'supporting cast' ingredient in dishes, but this shouldn't be the case! Simple, beautiful and delicious, these roasted red onion 'flowers' will steal the show at any meal.

17x
more quercetin is found in outer layers just beneath the skin **so don't over-peel**

SERVES 4
PREP TIME 5 MINUTES
COOK TIME 40 MINUTES

4 RED ONIONS
4 TBSP OLIVE OIL
2 TSP SMOKED SALT
1 TBSP THYME LEAVES, PLUS EXTRA TO GARNISH
FINELY GRATED ZEST OF 1 ORANGE, TO GARNISH

PREHEAT the oven to 200°C/Gas Mark 6.

SLICE the onions right down the centre into quarters or eighths, keeping intact the bottom 1cm of the bulb where the roots grow from.

ARRANGE the onions in a baking dish, brush them with the oil and sprinkle with the salt and thyme. Bake for 40 minutes until golden and tender.

SPRINKLE the onion 'flowers' with extra thyme and the orange zest and serve.

SPRING ONION POTATO PANCAKES

Growing up, these were one of my favourite lazy Sunday breakfast dishes when visiting my family in Malaysia. OK, the real deal is made with Chinese chives, but spring onions work just as well in this shamelessly Westernized recipe. Once cooked, the flavour mellows to a delicate, sweet richness to create moreish savoury pancakes that are nearly 50 per cent veg.

SERVES 4 (MAKES 12 PANCAKES)
PREP TIME 5 MINUTES
COOK TIME 10 MINUTES

- -

300G COLD LEFTOVER
MASHED POTATO

200G SPRING ONIONS, VERY
FINELY SLICED

2 EGGS

200ML MILK

50G PLAIN FLOUR

1 TSP BAKING POWDER

1 TSP MIXED SPICE

SALT AND PEPPER

OLIVE OIL, FOR FRYING

TO SERVE

100G CHERRY TOMATOES

4 FRIED EGGS

100G GRILLED MUSHROOMS

HANDFUL OF ROCKET

PINK PICKLED ONIONS WITH
LIME & BAY (SEE PAGE 64)

4x more phytonutrients are found in the leafy bits of **spring onions**

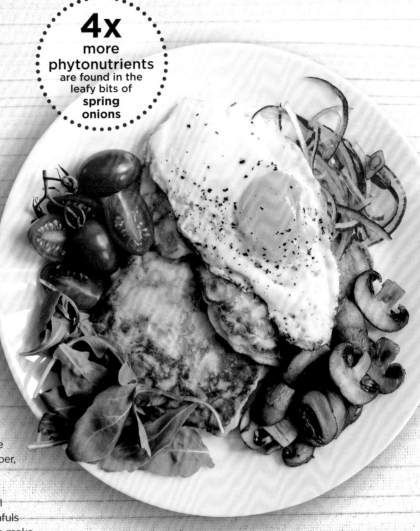

PLACE all the ingredients in a large bowl and season with salt and pepper, then mix until loosely combined.

GREASE a large frying pan with oil and heat until hot, then pour spoonfuls of the chunky batter into the pan to make small pancakes the size of a CD. Cook for about 1 minute on each side until cooked through. Remove from the pan and keep warm in a low oven until all the pancakes are made.

SERVE each portion of pancakes with cherry tomatoes, a fried egg, grilled mushrooms, a handful of rocket and some Pink Pickled Onions with Lime & Bay.

DON'T BIN THE BEST BIT

The green leafy bits of spring onions, and leeks for that matter, contain quadruple the beneficial compounds of the white stem according to researchers at The University of Life Sciences in Lublin, Poland. Yet these are precisely the bits most people end up binning. Simply don't over-peel and you will instantly boost nutrition.

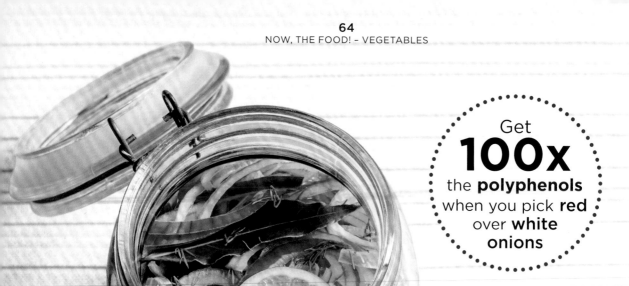

Get
100x
the **polyphenols**
when you pick **red**
over **white**
onions

PINK PICKLED ONIONS WITH LIME & BAY

Probably my favourite condiment in the whole world, these jewel-pink slivers
seem to work with pretty much everything, from a garnish on grilled chicken
or fish to great forkfuls stuffed in sandwiches.

MAKES ABOUT 200G

PREP TIME 10 MINUTES,
PLUS PICKLING

3 RED ONIONS, VERY THINLY SLICED

100ML CIDER VINEGAR

1 TBSP CASTER SUGAR

½ TSP SALT

1 LIME, THINLY SLICED

2 BAY LEAVES

A FEW DILL SPRIGS

PLACE all the ingredients in a non-reactive bowl
and toss together.

COVER and leave to infuse in the fridge for at
least 30 minutes or preferably overnight.

USE when infused or store the pickled onions in a
sterilized jar in the fridge for up to 3 months.

AJO BLANCO

This traditional southern Spanish soup's creamy almond base, sweet grape topping and icy serving temperature all conspire to take the harsh edge off an awful lot of raw garlic. Yes, I know it's a combination that sounds implausible (I admit I was highly sceptical before trying it too), but I promise you it just works. Oh boy, does it work.

SERVES 4

PREP TIME 15 MINUTES, PLUS CHILLING

3 GARLIC CLOVES, MINCED
200G FLAKED ALMONDS
100ML MILK
250ML WATER
2 TSP SALT
50ML EXTRA VIRGIN OLIVE OIL
2 TBSP SHERRY VINEGAR

TO SERVE
20G TOASTED FLAKED ALMONDS
HANDFUL OF GREEN GRAPES, HALVED
PAPRIKA

COMBINE all the ingredients except the oil and vinegar in a large bowl, cover and leave to chill in the fridge overnight.

BLITZ the soup in a food processor until smooth, then with the motor still running, drizzle in the oil and vinegar through the funnel. Add a little extra water if the soup is too thick.

PASS the soup through a sieve into a bowl, then cover and chill for at least 20 minutes until very cold.

LADLE the soup into bowls and serve topped with the flaked almonds, grapes and a sprinkling of paprika.

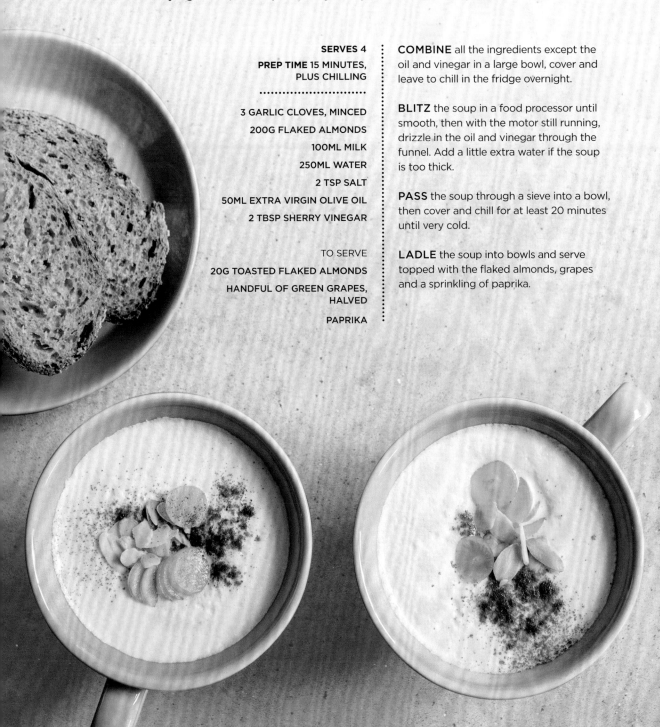

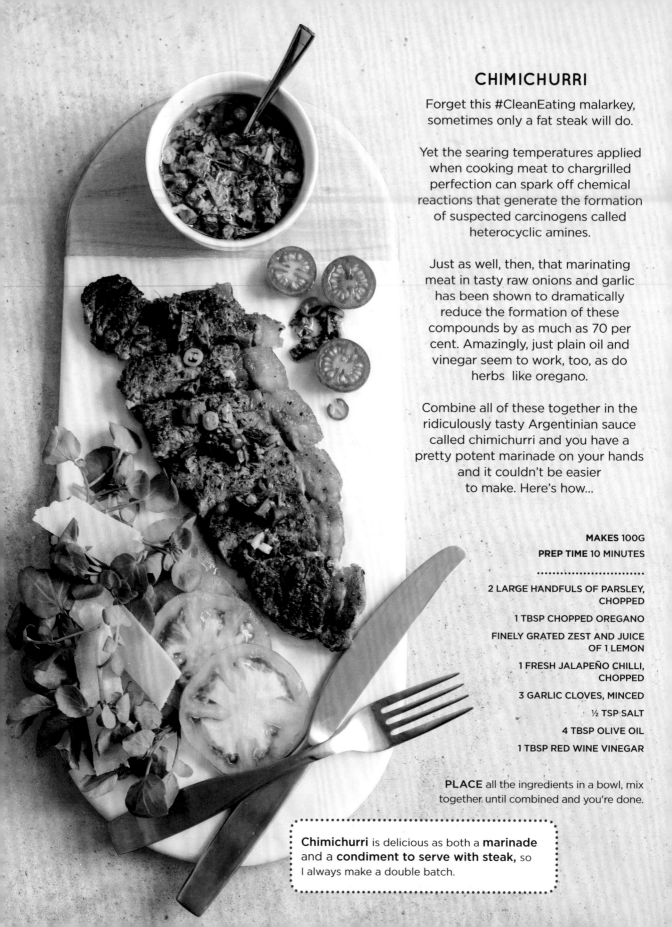

CHIMICHURRI

Forget this #CleanEating malarkey, sometimes only a fat steak will do.

Yet the searing temperatures applied when cooking meat to chargrilled perfection can spark off chemical reactions that generate the formation of suspected carcinogens called heterocyclic amines.

Just as well, then, that marinating meat in tasty raw onions and garlic has been shown to dramatically reduce the formation of these compounds by as much as 70 per cent. Amazingly, just plain oil and vinegar seem to work, too, as do herbs like oregano.

Combine all of these together in the ridiculously tasty Argentinian sauce called chimichurri and you have a pretty potent marinade on your hands and it couldn't be easier to make. Here's how...

MAKES 100G

PREP TIME 10 MINUTES

························

2 LARGE HANDFULS OF PARSLEY, CHOPPED

1 TBSP CHOPPED OREGANO

FINELY GRATED ZEST AND JUICE OF 1 LEMON

1 FRESH JALAPEÑO CHILLI, CHOPPED

3 GARLIC CLOVES, MINCED

½ TSP SALT

4 TBSP OLIVE OIL

1 TBSP RED WINE VINEGAR

PLACE all the ingredients in a bowl, mix together until combined and you're done.

> **Chimichurri** is delicious as both a **marinade** and a **condiment to serve with steak,** so I always make a double batch.

PEPPERS & CHILLIES

Both peppers and chillies are loaded with good stuff. In fact, red peppers were recently ranked the most antioxidant rich of the ten most commonly consumed veg in the Western diet according to a study at Cornell University – beating other nutritional heavyweights such as broccoli and spinach. A single 80g serving of peppers is packed with more than twice the vitamin C you need a day, plus a good helping of fibre, vitamin A and carotenoids. Add to this the growing stack of evidence behind the biological effects of the spicy chemical called capsaicin in chillies and you have a pretty potent nutritional cocktail on your hands.

 WEIGHT MANAGEMENT

A growing range of studies is beginning to point to the idea that eating chillies may not only be an effective way to control appetite, but also boost the number of calories you burn, while slowing the impact of carbs on your blood sugar. Too good to be true? Well, let's take a look at the evidence we have so far.

One small Dutch study published in the *International Journal of Obesity* decided to put the theory to the test by giving people just under 1g of dried chilli (about ½ teaspoon) half an hour before presenting them with giant, all-you-can-eat buffets at both lunch and dinner. Compared to those consuming a placebo, the chilli group slashed their total calorie consumption by about 15 per cent, while simultaneously reporting greater feelings of fullness. This sort of reduction is the equivalent to cutting out an impressive 240 calories per day – about the amount found in a chocolate bar – all without going hungry!

This trial echoed the findings of a series of Japanese studies, which found that chilli consumption not only reduces appetite, but also significantly increases the rate our bodies burn calories by raising our body temperature, especially after high-fat meals. Add this to the two small trials in Australia and South Africa that found supplementing chilli to a meal reduced the impact of that meal on blood sugar and I for one will be reaching for the hot sauce.

Is eating chillies the magic bullet to weight loss? Of course not. Could it be a tasty, nutritious way to potentially help manage weight in the context of a healthy diet? It seems it just might be! Let's see what future studies uncover. Watch this space.

 PARKINSON'S PREVENTION?

Observational studies have long noted the curious phenomenon that smokers have a much lower risk of developing Parkinson's disease – in fact, as much as 50 per cent less. Even non-smokers regularly exposed to cigarette smoke tend to have a lower incidence of the debilitating illness, a phenomenon that some researchers have attributed to the nicotine the fumes contain. The only problem here is the *massive* increased risk of developing heart disease and cancer in smokers, which obviously vastly outweighs any potential health benefits. But, crazy as it sounds, could there be a way to get hold of some of nicotine's potential benefits in a safe way? Maybe even through diet?

This question piqued the interest of researchers at the University of Washington who noted that tiny amounts of nicotine are also found in relatives of the tobacco plant that just happen to be popular food crops, namely tomatoes, potatoes, peppers and aubergines. When I say tiny, generous consumption of these foods could provide about two-millionths of a gram of nicotine in the average daily diet – hundreds of times less than smoking itself. Yet this amount is similar to that which passive smokers experience in a smoke-filled room over a few hours – so could it have an effect? The Washingtonians compared the diets of hundreds of recently diagnosed patients with Parkinson's to a control group. They found that while consuming comparatively low-nicotine foods such as potatoes and aubergines made no difference, eating higher-nicotine foods like peppers (which contain five times that of spuds) was correlated with a significantly lower risk of developing Parkinson's.

In fact, those who ate peppers daily showed half the risk of those who never ate them at all. Intriguing. Of course, this sort of study simply shows a correlation, not causation. It might well be one of the many other chemicals in peppers that is responsible. Maybe a combination of several? In fact, it might not be the peppers at all, just something people who eat lots of peppers tend to do – like, say, eating lots of vegetables generally. Much more research would need to be done before we know for sure, but in the meantime popping slices of smoky-sweet roast peppers into any dish I can fit them into is hardly a chore.

HIGHEST CAROTENES

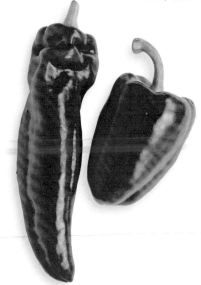

7,137 carotenes (mg/g)

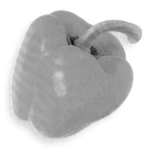

5,293 carotenes (mg/g)

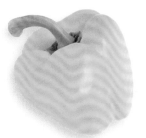

2,236 carotenes (mg/g)

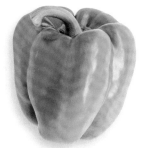

1,514 carotenes (mg/g)

LOWEST CAROTENES

REACH FOR RED

As with pretty much all fruit and veg, the evidence shows that the brighter their colour, the more phytonutrients peppers contain. This means that ripe red peppers can boast as much as five times the polyphenols *and* carotenes of the immature green kind, with the fruit also accumulating tasty sugars and aroma compounds as they redden. What a deal. What about yellow and orange ones? These are just cultivars that naturally accumulate fewer carotene pigments, meaning they never turn quite as red (or nutrient dense) as the others.

ROAST BEATS RAW

Good news! As with other crops rich in carotenes (think tomatoes and, well, carrots) most studies suggest that cooking improves the polyphenol content of peppers by as much as twice their raw content. And the food science geeks have gone one step further, investigating the impact of different cooking techniques on the nutritional content of chillies and peppers, from boiling (who on earth boils peppers?), to steaming, grilling, roasting, stir-frying and microwaving. As usual, dry-heat cooking methods retain most nutrients by not only preventing the leaching of nutrients into cooking water, but also concentrating levels of the good stuff in the veg as it cooks down. When you concentrate phytonutrients, you conveniently also concentrate sugars, acids and aroma compounds, making for tastier results, so go for baked, roasted and grilled every time.

You'd have to eat nearly **5 green peppers** to get as many phytonutrients as just **1 red one**

DON'T BIN THE WHITE STUFF!

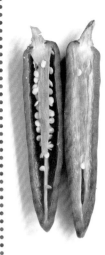

You know that white spongy tissue on the inside of chillies and peppers? The stuff around the seeds that's a fiddle to remove? Well don't! Not only will you instantly dispense with a chore, but you just might get more nutrition as a result. In one Mexican study, scientists found that this white stuff in peppers, which us plant geeks call the 'placenta', contains the highest concentrations of antioxidants and polyphenols – as much as four times that of the flesh itself. I love when being lazy pays off.

BE A JAR HEAD

There are a few great brands of jarred roasted peppers out there that contain nothing other than peppers, a little salt and a dose of antioxidants as a natural preservative, meaning you get super-convenient nutrition at the twist of a lid. These can seem pricey when compared to other jarred veg, however, and because I am a terrible cheapskate I carried out a price comparison. I bought and roasted a whole bunch of fresh supermarket 'value' red peppers and compared the results weight-for-weight with the contents of a jar. And guess what? Even the fanciest jars of smoky Spanish peppers are half the price of roasting your own and – if you get a good brand – have a flavour that's surprisingly just as good. Go for the brightest red ones you can find, not the faded orangey types, for maximum carotene kick.

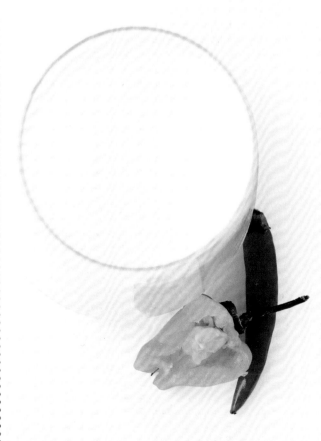

HANDLING THE HEAT

Interested in the benefits of chillies, but don't like your food volcano-strength? Fortunately, there are things you can do about this. A fat-loving protein in milk called casein works essentially like detergent to stop the capsaicin binding with the pain receptors on your tongue – thereby reducing their burn. It has to be actual milk, though (goats' milk is fine too), just not soya, almond or coconut. What has even more casein than milk? Well, cheese, which in many ways is essentially milk with some of the water removed. Paired with some cooling cottage cheese or even thick Greek yogurt, even the super-strength chillies can taste surprisingly mild.

Dried chilli flakes have the capsaicin trapped within their fibrous structures, meaning it can take a while for these to leach out and become detectable on your tongue. I have found you can sprinkle on a surprising amount of these at the table without noticing a huge difference, yet take an identical quantity and add it to the same dish as it simmers on the stove and it'll blow your head off. Moral of the story? Sprinkle, don't simmer.

Finally, it is worth noting that scientific trials have demonstrated that tolerance to capsaicin can be acquired extremely rapidly. In as little as 5 days, what was once an excruciating burn can be barely noticeable with a daily exposure. So try upping your dose a little each day and see how you go.

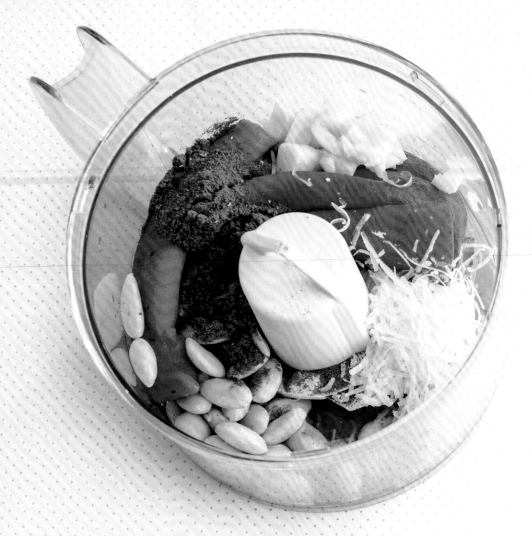

MOJO PICÓN

This thick, smoky roasted pepper sauce from the Canary Islands can be whizzed up in seconds and used as a super-healthy, super-quick alternative to regular tomato sauce – on pizzas, in sandwiches or pasta, even as a grown-up take on tomato ketchup.

MAKES 250G

PREP TIME 5 MINUTES

....

400G JAR ROASTED RED PEPPERS

2 GARLIC CLOVES, SLICED

1 TBSP SMOKED PAPRIKA

1 TBSP GRATED PARMESAN CHEESE

100G WHOLE ALMONDS

1 TBSP RED WINE VINEGAR

4 TBSP OLIVE OIL

BLITZ all the ingredients together in a food processor until smooth.

USE immediately or store the sauce in the fridge for up to 1 week.

HOW TO SERVE

(1) PASTA SAUCE

Mojo Picón makes the world's best pasta sauce, even if I do say so myself! Toss it through some hot **wholegrain fusilli or penne** and serve topped with a few **fresh basil leaves** and a dusting of grated **Parmesan cheese**. Pop it in a plastic container, give it a quick zap in the office microwave and you have an instant super-healthy workday lunch to scoff al desko.

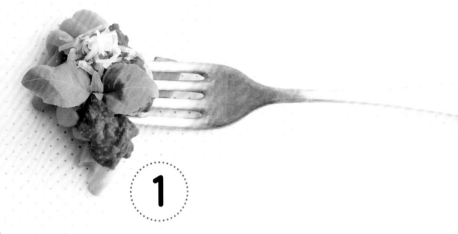

1

(2) SANDWICH TOPPING

For a super-fast weekday dinner, spread the sauce thickly over freshly toasted **wholegrain sourdough**, top with chunky slices of **avocado** and scatter crunchy **pistachios**, crumbled **feta cheese** and thinly sliced **red onions** over the top.

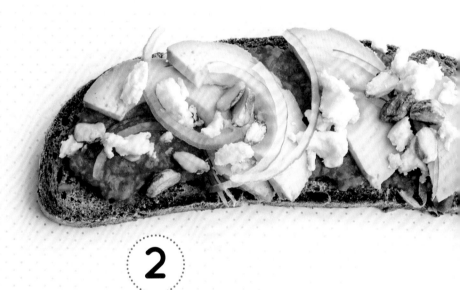

2

(3) PIZZA TOPPING

Getting kids to eat their 5-a-day can be tricky, but disguising those vegetables in the form of a pizza can be an ingeniously sneaky way to get children to enjoying salad by stealth. Spread the Mojo Picón over a **wholegrain pitta**, top with some slices of leftover **cooked chicken**, a couple of extra **veggies** and a few shavings of **Parmesan cheese**, then place on a baking sheet and cook under a preheated medium grill for 5 minutes. Here I have used **cherry tomatoes** and a bit of **rocket**, but more kid-friendly vegetables like sweetcorn, carrots and peas will work just as well.

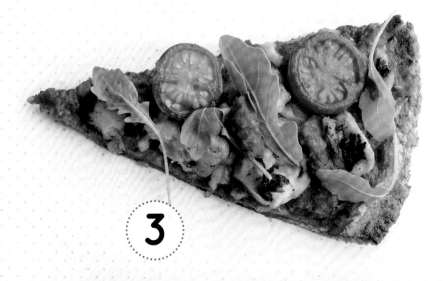

3

SPICY FRITTATA MUFFINS

These savoury, high-protein muffins, packed with veggies, are great as a grab-as-you-run-out-the-door breakfast or lunch-box treat. They even freeze beautifully, too. The protein in eggs tempers the perception of spicy flavours, meaning you can add a lot more chilli than other recipes, without it blowing your head off.

MAKES 12 MUFFINS
PREP TIME 15 MINUTES
COOK TIME 20 MINUTES

OLIVE OIL, FOR GREASING
6 EGGS, BEATEN
4 TBSP GREEK YOGURT
1 TSP MIXED SPICE
6 TBSP POLENTA OR CORNMEAL
4 TBSP FINELY GRATED PARMESAN CHEESE, PLUS EXTRA FOR SPRINKLING
1 TSP RED CHILLI FLAKES
50G CARROT, GRATED
100G FROZEN SWEETCORN
3 SPRING ONIONS, CUT INTO SMALL ROUNDS
100G COURGETTE, CUT INTO SMALL CUBES
150G SWEET POTATO, GRATED
1 TSP BAKING POWDER
SALT AND PEPPER

TO GARNISH
1 RED CHILLI, THINLY SLICED
1 TSP CHOPPED DILL

PREHEAT the oven to 180°C/Gas Mark 4 and grease the sections of a 12-hole muffin tray with oil or line them with paper muffin cases.

PLACE all the ingredients in a large bowl, season generously with salt and pepper and mix together until combined.

POUR the mixture into the prepared muffin holes, then sprinkle the muffins with a little extra Parmesan.

BAKE for 20 minutes. Remove the muffins from the tray immediately to prevent them from going soggy and transfer to a wire rack to cool.

SERVE the muffins warm or cold, sprinkled with extra Parmesan, sliced chillies and dill.

The world's hottest chilli, the **Carolina Reaper**, can contain more capsaicin than pepper spray

WEAPONS-GRADE SPICE

Chillies evolved the ability to produce spicy capsaicin as a defence against mammals, to deter them from coming along and scoffing the fruit and destroying the plant's all-important seeds as they pass through their digestive tracts.

So why do the plants spend all that energy making a fleshy, eye-catching, otherwise tasty fruit? Well, the answer is that in the wild chillies use birds to disperse their seeds. Avian digestive tracts are harmless to chilli seeds, allowing them to pass through unscathed and spread far and wide. You see, capsaicin does not affect birds at all, it's a selective deterrent that puts off foes but is undetectable to friends. Plants are endlessly fascinating.

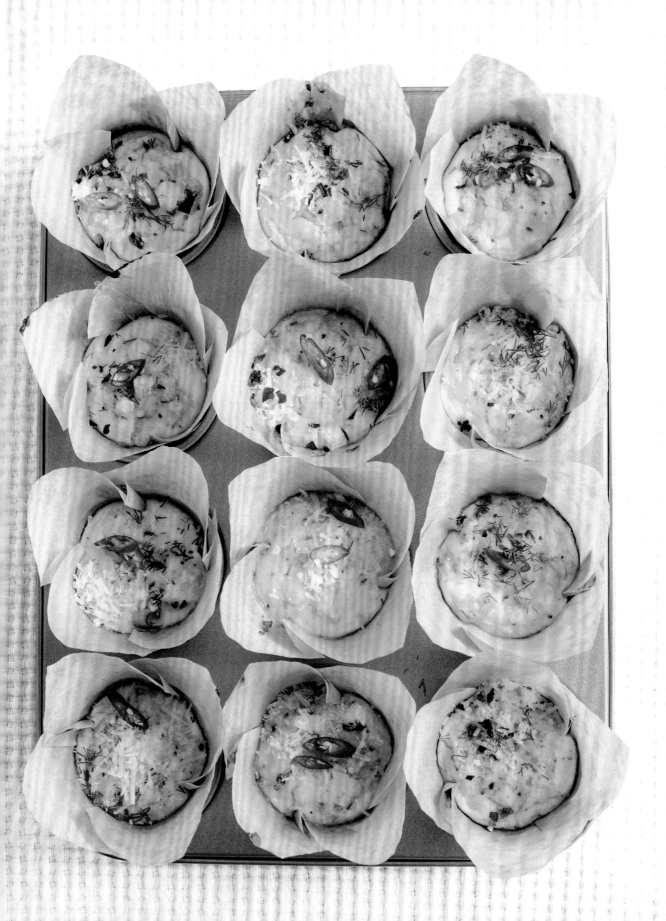

BLUEBERRY & CHILLI CHEESE TOASTIE

Capsaicin is fat soluble and tempered by the effect of a protein called casein in milk. This makes a good old cheese toastie the ideal delivery vehicle for the healthy chilli payload. This veggie-enhanced recipe makes a perfect quick lunch with a leafy side salad and crunchy apple.

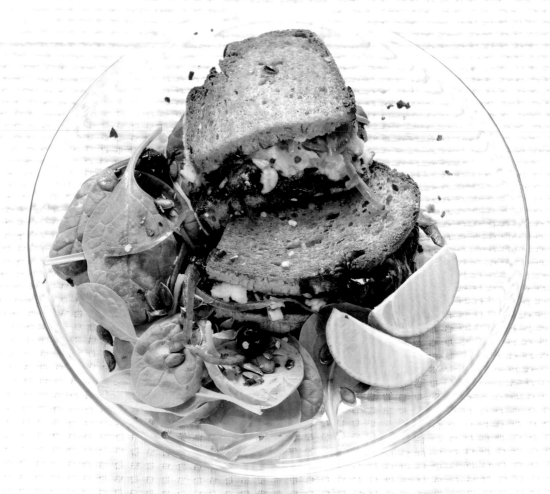

SERVES 1

PREP TIME 10 MINUTES

COOK TIME 4 MINUTES

....

1 TBSP 5-MINUTE BLUEBERRY COMPOTE (SEE PAGE 128)

1 TSP BALSAMIC VINEGAR

1 TSP RED CHILLI FLAKES

2 SLICES OF SOURDOUGH BREAD

A FEW SLICES OF RED ONION

50G MATURE CHEDDAR CHEESE, SLICED

SMALL HANDFUL OF SPINACH LEAVES

OLIVE OIL, FOR FRYING

MIX the blueberry compote, balsamic vinegar and chilli flakes together in a small bowl.

ASSEMBLE the sandwich, filling the sourdough slices with the red onion, cheese, spinach and blueberry mixture.

HEAT a little oil in a frying pan, carefully add the sandwich and toast over a low heat for 2 minutes on each side, turning once, until golden.

INSTANT CHOCOLATE-CHILLI 'ICE CREAM'

OK, I'll admit it, this is not really an ice cream at all. But despite its improbably healthy ingredients and lazy preparation, this stuff really does work as a deliciously fresh, less cloying alternative to the full-fat stuff on hot summer days. The ice-cold temperature knocks back the fire power of the chilli flakes, meaning you can add loads more than you might think.

SERVES 2

PREP TIME 10 MINUTES

....

2 VERY RIPE BANANAS, FROZEN

1 TSP GRANULATED STEVIA (BAKING BLEND)

½ TSP VANILLA EXTRACT

1 TSP PEANUT BUTTER

½ TSP RED CHILLI FLAKES

1 TBSP NATURAL COCOA POWDER

TO DECORATE

CHOPPED NUTS (I USED PISTACHIOS)

FRESH FRUIT (I MADE A BANANA SPLIT WITH CHERRIES)

DARK CHOCOLATE CHIPS

2 TSP WHIPPED CREAM

BLITZ all the ingredients together in a food processor until smooth.

DECORATE with the chopped nuts, fresh fruit, chocolate chips and whipped cream and serve immediately.

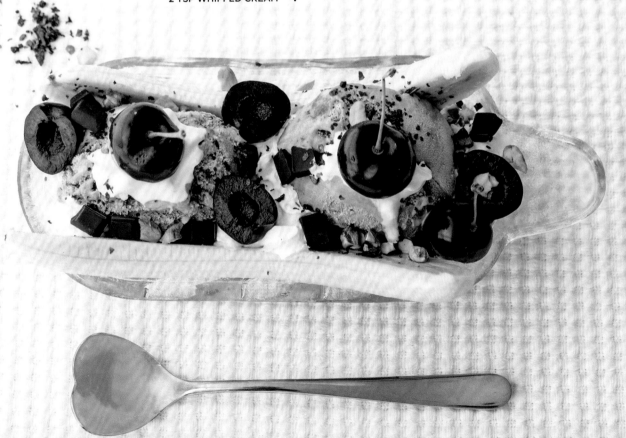

WORLD'S EASIEST CHILLI SAUCE

During my research into chillies, I stumbled across a fascinating trial by the University of Tasmania that found that adding chillies to people's everyday diet, in the form of a basic chilli sauce, could significantly reduce their spikes of insulin after a meal. The best bit? They even gave the rough formula for the proportions of chilli, sugar, onion, vinegar and salt they used. In their introduction they also happened to list other spices, including garlic, turmeric and cinnamon, which had previously been shown to have beneficial effects on digestive function and fat metabolism. Why not bung them all together? I did, and with surprisingly delicious consequences. Ladies and gents, I give you the world's easiest (and tastiest) hot sauce.

MAKES 1 X 500ML JAR

PREP TIME 10 MINUTES, PLUS STEEPING

• •

1 RED ONION, SLICED

3 GARLIC CLOVES, MINCED

THUMB-SIZED PIECE OF FRESH ROOT GINGER, PEELED AND SLICED

THUMB-SIZED PIECE OF FRESH TURMERIC, PEELED AND SLICED, OR 2 TSP TURMERIC POWDER

½ TSP CINNAMON

FINELY GRATED ZEST OF 2 LEMONS

2 TSP BLACK PEPPERCORNS

2 TSP SALT

2 TBSP CLEAR HONEY

150G RED CHILLIES, SLICED (BUT DON'T BOTHER TO DESEED)

1 THYME SPRIG

ABOUT 200ML CIDER VINEGAR

PACK all the ingredients except the vinegar as tightly as possible into a sterilized 500ml Kilner or jam jar, then fill to the brim with the vinegar, ensuring all the ingredients are submerged.

SEAL the jar and leave it to steep in a cool, dark place for 1 week.

WHEN ready, transfer the mixture to a food processor and blitz until smooth. This stuff goes with anything and will keep in a sealable jar or glass bottle in the fridge for up to 6 months.

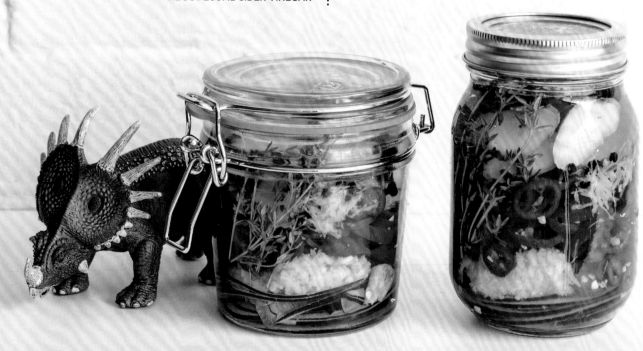

ASPARAGUS

Like most greens, asparagus is a real nutritional superstar, packing a hefty dose of vitamins A, C, K and folate into the tasty spears. It is a rich source of a polyphenol called rutin, too, which research suggests may help reduce inflammation, blood pressure and cholesterol and improve circulation. Add to that a generous amount of fibre, including prebiotic inulin, which feeds colonies of friendly gut bacteria linked to a reduced incidence of cancer and an enhanced immune function, and asparagus stacks up as a pretty great nutritional all-rounder. Here's how to eat it at its very best.

 ## GO FOR GREEN

From wispy green tips to stalks as fat as your thumb, pale ivory spears to stems of dazzling purple, asparagus comes in loads of forms. As always, simply popping one type over another into your shopping basket can make a significant nutritional difference. Here is the run down.

Purple

By now I am sure you will have got used to me banging on about purple anthocyanin pigments and how the red and purple varieties of regular crops that contain them are almost always far higher in phytonutrients as a result. Key word: *almost* – in the case of purple asparagus, there appears to be a negligible difference. Although one Japanese study showed that it can have 4 per cent more polyphenols than regular green asparagus, a US study published just a year later, which assessed more than double the number of varieties, found that purple had 10 per cent *fewer* polyphenols and antioxidants than green. Hardly earth-shattering stats either way, and as purple tends to lose its pretty hue when cooked there is probably little meaningful difference between the two, other than the 'fancy factor' price tag, of course!

White

These snowy spears aren't a different genetic variety, but regular green asparagus that has been grown in the dark by simply piling mounds of soil on top of the plants. The absence of UV rays causes the stems to become far more tender in texture (i.e. lower in healthy fibre) and delicate in flavour (i.e. contain fewer tasty polyphenols).

As a consequence, studies across the board show that white asparagus can contain as little as half the polyphenols of green asparagus, with rutin levels so low they were undetectable. As if that wasn't bad enough for the poor pallid guys, bog-standard green spears also appear to be significantly higher in pretty much every essential vitamin and mineral, including 50 per cent more calcium, twice the vitamins B and C and zinc, and a massive 20 times the vitamin A. So, if it's health benefits you are after, get green every time.

Green asparagus has

2x

the **polyphenols** and **vitamins B** and **C** of **white asparagus**

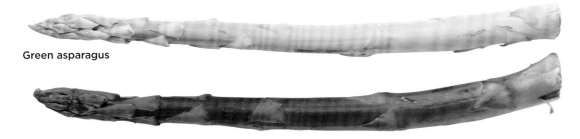

Green asparagus

Purple asparagus

White asparagus

PICK THE LONG & LANKY

The asparagus we eat are the young shoots of the plant that erupt from underground each spring, capable of growing at an astonishing rate. But what happens to the nutritional content of these shoots amid all the furious chemical reactions fuelling their growth? Well, we didn't really know until a Japanese team put it to the test. They found that the heart-healthy rutin content increased exponentially as the stems grew, meaning stems 24cm long had twice that of the stubby 8cm ones that were just a week or two younger.

As the stalks lengthen they also tend to become skinnier, greatly increasing the surface area of each spear where rutin is concentrated. This betrays rutin's function in plants as a biological sunscreen, whose antioxidant effect protects their cells from UV damage (which explains why there is next to none in spears grown in the dark). Pick the cheaper stems sold at pencil thickness instead of the 'premium' ones the width of your finger and you can get double the rutin, gram for gram, according to a trial at Canada's University of Guelph, and at a lower cost to boot.

EAT IT ASAP

Being packed with rapidly growing cells, asparagus spears quickly start burning up the sugars they contain from the second they are harvested. In fact, within just a week (the amount of time it can take to get from farm to store) they can be literally half as sweet and significantly tougher in texture, not to mention having far less vitamin C. Although, thankfully, rutin levels remain pretty stable over time, for the best possible flavour buy asparagus spears with the longest expiry date and eat them as soon as you get home.

There is 100% more of the antioxidant rutin in skinnier spears

COOKED OR RAW?

As with many greens, cooking asparagus can spike its nutritional value, bumping up its levels of polyphenols and vitamins – we are talking a 25 per cent boost in its levels of a host of powerful antioxidants like betacarotene, lutein (see page 94) and quercetin (see page 58), and a massive doubling of its rutin content after a few minutes in a pan. In fact, in an exhaustive study of the impact of different cooking methods on 20 different vegetables, a team at Spain's University of Murcia found that asparagus was one of the only crops to see no appreciable decrease in antioxidant activity in any cooking method, including boiling, baking, microwaving, griddling or frying. So, enjoy it however you fancy!

There is only one downside to cooking asparagus, however, and that is that it effectively halves its levels of prebiotics like inulin, which can help boost the levels of friendly bacteria in your gut. This is a shame as, gram for gram, asparagus is one of the best sources of these indigestible carbs per serving among everyday foods – alongside cooked onions, artichokes and wholemeal bread. Although I was initially sceptical, I was pleasantly surprised to find that the raw stuff also has a much sweeter flavour and delicious crunch.

So what's the take-away here? Eat this delicious, super-versatile veg any way you like, and if you'd like some inspiration on trying it raw there's a great recipe for an asparagus salad (even if I do say so myself) on the opposite page.

AFTER-EFFECTS

Asparagus contains asparagusic acid, a sulphur-based compound that our bodies break down into chemicals that can impart a characteristic whiff of garlic or cooked cabbage to your pee as little as an hour or two after eating it. Strangely, this does not appear to be a universal phenomenon, however. In fact, the world seems to be divided into four groups of people: those who produce more odour and those who produce less, and those who can smell it and those who can't, meaning you might *think* it doesn't make your pee smell even if it really, really does.

Yes, serious scientists have actually investigated this, in over half a dozen different studies in Britain, France and the United States. Although being able to detect the smell has been linked to genetics, we still have really no idea what causes some people to mysteriously not produce the smell in the first place. Boy, that is one study I am glad I am not running!

JAPANESE SHAVED ASPARAGUS SALAD

My whole life I wanted to go to Japan. Not just for the culture, landscapes or even the amazing plants, but for the food. Oh the food. But what took me by surprise a few years back when I was lucky enough to be filming there, was that my favourite dish was not some fancy sushi or trendy fusion ramen, but a simple salad in a roadside restaurant. This is my attempt to recreate it.

SERVES 2

PREP TIME 10 MINUTES

....

200G ASPARAGUS

SMALL HANDFUL OF GREEN BEANS, ABOUT 50G, HALVED

1 RED CHICORY, LEAVES SEPARATED

SMALL HANDFUL OF MANGETOUT, ABOUT 50G, HALVED

DRESSING

2 TBSP GARLIC MAYONNAISE

1 TBSP TAHINI

1 TSP SOY SAUCE

1 TSP SUGAR

¼ TSP SALT

FINELY GRATED ZEST AND JUICE OF ½ LEMON

CUT off the tips of the asparagus and set aside, then slice the rest of the stems into thin ribbons using a vegetable peeler.

ARRANGE the asparagus tips and ribbons on a plate with the remaining vegetables.

COMBINE all the dressing ingredients together in a small bowl, then drizzle over the salad and serve.

Eat raw for

DOUBLE

the **gut-friendly prebiotics**

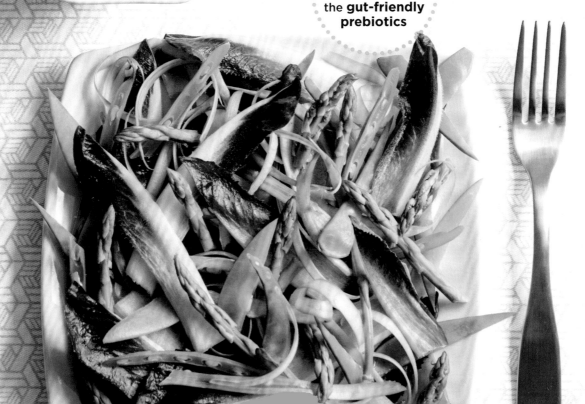

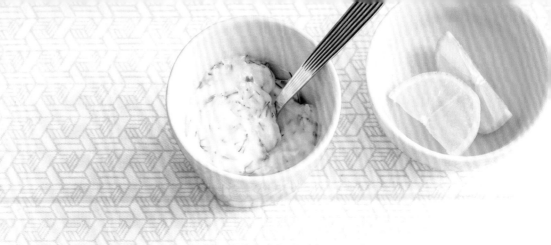

ROAST ASPARAGUS & SALMON WITH HERB MAYO

Bung a bunch of things in a tin and bake it. Get a complete (and über-healthy) meal in about 30 minutes. That's my kind of cooking.

SERVES 4
PREP TIME 10 MINUTES
COOK TIME 15–20 MINUTES

· · · · · · · · · · · · · · · · · · · ·

1 TSP HORSERADISH
2 GARLIC CLOVES, CRUSHED
2 TBSP OLIVE OIL
FINELY GRATED ZEST OF 1 LEMON
4 SALMON STEAKS, ABOUT 150G EACH
400G ASPARAGUS
1 LEMON, SLICED
400G CHERRY TOMATOES
SALT AND PEPPER

HERB MAYO
4 TBSP MAYONNAISE
1 TBSP MILK
1 TBSP CHOPPED DILL
1 TSP CHOPPED PARSLEY
3 SPRING ONIONS, CHOPPED

TO SERVE
1 LARGE BUNCH OF WATERCRESS
LEMON WEDGES

PREHEAT the oven to 200°C/Gas Mark 6.

MIX the horseradish, garlic, olive oil and lemon zest together in a small bowl.

LAY the salmon steaks in the centre of a large baking sheet with the asparagus, lemon slices and tomatoes. Brush the salmon and vegetables with the oil mixture and season well. Bake for 15–20 minutes, or until the fish is cooked through and the asparagus is tender.

MEANWHILE, blitz all the herb mayo ingredients together in a food processor to make a smooth sauce.

DIVIDE the salmon and vegetables among 4 serving plates, then add a small bunch of watercress and a dollop of the herb mayo to each one. Serve with lemon wedges for squeezing over.

This tastes even better with a pile of my **Pink Pickled Onions with Lime & Bay** (see page 64).

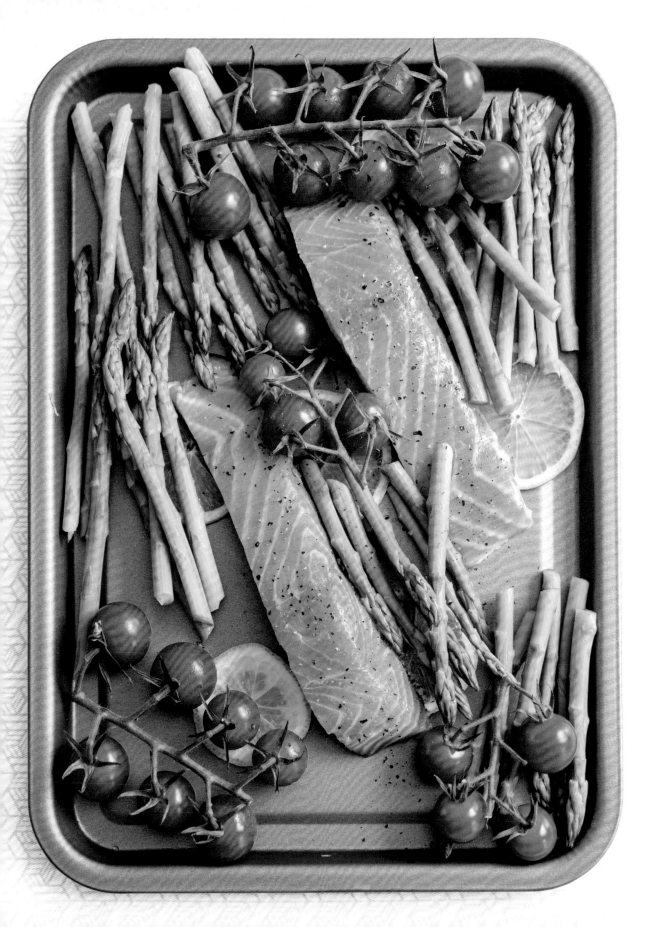

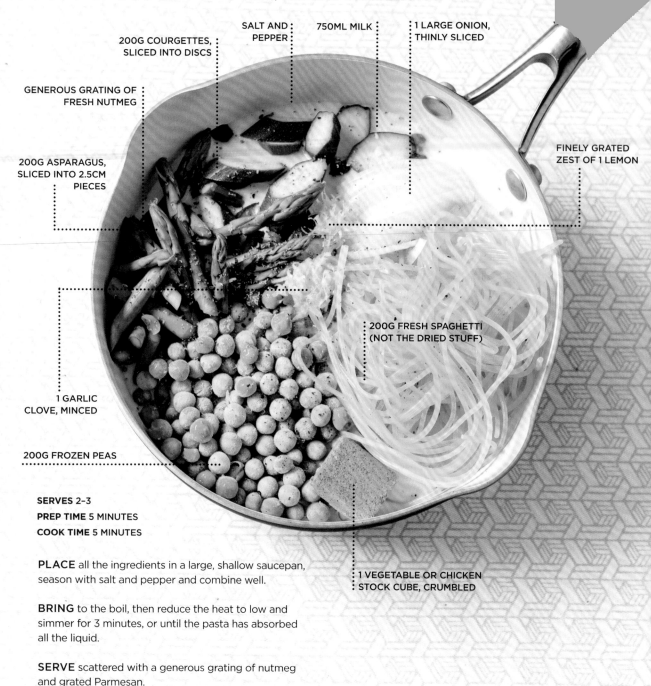

200G COURGETTES, SLICED INTO DISCS

SALT AND PEPPER

750ML MILK

1 LARGE ONION, THINLY SLICED

GENEROUS GRATING OF FRESH NUTMEG

FINELY GRATED ZEST OF 1 LEMON

200G ASPARAGUS, SLICED INTO 2.5CM PIECES

200G FRESH SPAGHETTI (NOT THE DRIED STUFF)

1 GARLIC CLOVE, MINCED

200G FROZEN PEAS

1 VEGETABLE OR CHICKEN STOCK CUBE, CRUMBLED

SERVES 2–3
PREP TIME 5 MINUTES
COOK TIME 5 MINUTES

PLACE all the ingredients in a large, shallow saucepan, season with salt and pepper and combine well.

BRING to the boil, then reduce the heat to low and simmer for 3 minutes, or until the pasta has absorbed all the liquid.

SERVE scattered with a generous grating of nutmeg and grated Parmesan.

5-MINUTE PASTA PRIMAVERA

As you probably know by now, I love me a one-pot pasta recipe, but this has to be my favourite of them all. Fast, healthy food at its best, using fresh spaghetti from the chiller counter means the whole lot cooks in 5 minutes or less, sauce and all. Containing three times more veggies than it does pasta, this is a dish full of flavour, not stodgy carbs.

BEETROOT

Beets have experienced a meteoric rise in popularity in the last few years undoubtedly fuelled, at least in part, by the huge hype surrounding emerging evidence that links a compound called dietary nitrate, which beets are particularly rich in, with a range of potential health benefits. Having trouble separating fact from fiction? Here's an impartial take on the latest evidence surrounding the almighty beetroot.

BLOOD PRESSURE

A range of trials has demonstrated that the dietary nitrate found in beetroot can help relax arteries, causing these vessels to widen and therefore reduce the pressure of the blood flowing through them. For example, in a small but influential trial funded by the British Heart Foundation, patients with raised blood pressure who drank a 250ml glass of beetroot juice every day saw a decrease of as much as 8/4mmHg within just 4 weeks of consumption. This was enough to bring many of these hypertensives back to within the 'normal' range, all with zero reported side-effects. A fall on a par with that seen with a standard dose of some prescription drugs! This 8-point fall in systolic blood pressure is relevant because every 2-point *rise* is thought to increase the risk of heart disease and stroke by approximately 10 per cent.

These falls were observed despite the fact that half the group were already taking blood-pressure drugs, suggesting beetroot juice could further lower hypertension in people who had already seen an improvement with medication. In fact, the authors even postulated that this effect 'may be greater in patients with more severe hypertension' – some seriously positive-sounding findings. While they were also very quick to point out that much longer trials with far more people are needed before beetroot juice becomes recognized (or refuted) as a valid treatment, this trial is just one of more than a dozen studies in the last decade that consistently suggest dietary nitrate consumption in the form of beetroot juice could help maintain and even modestly reduce high blood pressure. This is a good excuse for a smoothie if ever there was one.

ATHLETIC PERFORMANCE

Evidence from all over the world is beginning to point to the idea that beetroot consumption can also boost athletic performance. Chuck a bunch of blokes on bikes and they could pedal for 16 per cent longer just 3 hours after drinking a couple of glasses of beetroot juice, according to the Swiss Institute of Sports Medicine. Do the same thing with rugby players and they sprint a far more modest 3.5 per cent faster and even make decisions 3 per cent more quickly, says the University of Exeter. Across the board, it appears that beetroot's impact on exercise stamina is much greater than the only very slight improvement in speed or intensity, according to a well-conducted review of 17 studies by the University of Sydney. So, gym bunnies, beets might allow you to stay on the treadmill a few minutes longer, but when it comes to speed they'll probably only make a noticeable benefit if you are an elite athlete looking to 'beet' the competition by a second or two.

IMPROVING QUALITY OF LIFE

The vast majority of the population aren't Olympians, so frankly who cares about shaving seconds off a race time? Well, it turns out these effects may be even greater in the inactive, which may hold promise for people whose fitness level greatly limits their everyday activities. Older patients with peripheral arterial disease (PAD), for example, have poor blood flow to their legs, which can make walking for just a few minutes excruciating. Give them a large (500ml) glass of beetroot juice, according to a small trial at Duke University Medical Center, North Carolina, however, and they can walk comfortably for 18 per cent longer, with the juice significantly improving the oxygen supply to their calf muscles. The extent of this improvement was roughly a third that experienced by patients after 3 months of physio – but kicked in just *3 hours* after drinking the juice.

Similar results have also been seen in patients with degenerative lung disease and heart failure, with up to an astonishing 24 per cent improvement in exercise endurance reported by two small trials at Wake Forest University in the United States. This *could* make a massive potential difference to someone's quality of life in exchange for just a couple of glasses of juice, so it might well be a habit worth taking up while we wait for the results of more research to come in.

🧺 BEST OF THE BEST

Amid all this booming research interest in dietary nitrate there has been surprisingly little work done to assess which of the hundreds of varieties of beetroot worldwide contain the heftiest doses. The one study I could find reported a whopping eightfold difference between the amounts of dietary nitrate in a group of local varieties in Upper Austria, so this clearly could make a big difference. I guess for non-Austrians, we will just have to wait and see!

However, there is more to beetroot than nitrate. In fact, in the antioxidant stakes it ranks among the highest of anything in the veg aisle, right up there with spinach, Brussels sprouts and kale, according to a study by Cornell University. What's more, the vivid red compounds behind this activity (known as betalains) are unusual in the plant kingdom, with beetroot essentially being the only common dietary source. Very early research in test tubes and animals suggests that these may reduce inflammation, protect cells from DNA damage, reduce the oxidation of 'bad' LDL cholesterol (a risk factor for heart disease) and even boost your body's own defence mechanisms against carcinogenic chemicals. Intriguing!

The best bit? As these are pigments, you can judge how rich your beets are in betalains at a mere glance: the redder the flesh, the more antioxidant activity they are likely to contain, according to Poznań University of Natural Sciences in Poland. White beetroots have essentially no betalains, with the pretty candy-striped ones only containing tiny amounts of the pigment in their powder-pink rings. Yellow beets are given their golden hue by a different form of betalain with a far lower antioxidant capacity, meaning that only red beets were a good indicator of this potential. Go for deep red or purple every time.

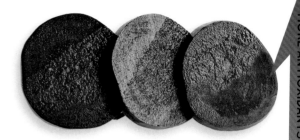

Red Ace

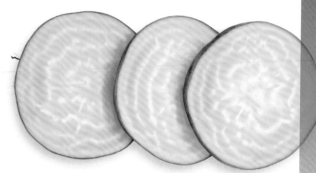

Burpees Golden

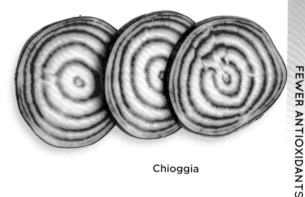

Chioggia

MORE ANTIOXIDANTS

FEWER ANTIOXIDANTS

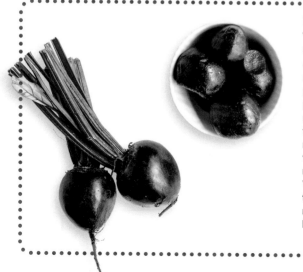

EMBRACE LAZINESS

OK, I'll admit it. I'm lazy in the kitchen. I rarely buy fresh beetroots, especially when precooked, vacuum-sealed packs are often far more readily available in my local supermarket for the same price or cheaper. So I was delighted to find that processed beets possess not only much more antioxidant activity than raw, but also more potentially heart-healthy betalains than cooking your own from scratch, according to the Berlin University of Technology. The researchers tried boiling, roasting, microwaving and commercial vacuum-cooking beetroot and found across the board all methods caused its antioxidant activity to double or even triple. When the same tests were run on betalain pigments, they found that although boiling and roasting lead to slight decreases, microwaving and vacuum-cooking actually caused these to rise by as much as 20 per cent. Hooray for kitchen short cuts!

ULTIMATE BEET BURGERS

Smoky, rich and packed with umami – I'm no vegetarian, but I would pick these over the beef version any day. Wholesome and healthy, without any sacrificing of flavour.

MAKES 4 BURGERS
PREP TIME 20 MINUTES,
PLUS SOAKING AND CHILLING
COOK TIME 45 MINUTES

....

100G DRIED SLICED SHIITAKE MUSHROOMS
250G COOKED BEETROOT, CUBED
1 SMALL ONION, FINELY SLICED
2 TBSP OLIVE OIL, PLUS EXTRA FOR FRYING
100G PITTED BLACK OLIVES, SLICED
1 TSP BLACK PEPPER
2 GARLIC CLOVES, FINELY CHOPPED
1 TBSP SMOKED PAPRIKA
1 VEGETABLE STOCK CUBE, CRUMBLED
100G COOKED BROWN RICE
1 EGG, BEATEN
1 SLICE OF STALE WHOLEGRAIN BREAD, TORN INTO CRUMBS
250G DRAINED AND RINSED CANNED BLACK BEANS

TO SERVE
4 WHOLEGRAIN BURGER BUNS
2 TOMATOES, SLICED
GRATED CHEDDAR CHEESE
SLICED AVOCADO
ROCKET LEAVES
PINK PICKLED ONIONS WITH LIME & BAY (SEE PAGE 64)

PREHEAT the oven to 200°C/Gas Mark 6. Place the mushrooms in a heatproof bowl, pour over hot water and leave to soak for 10 minutes. Drain and discard the soaking liquid.

COMBINE the mushrooms, beetroot and onion in a bowl, then tip into a roasting tin and toss with the oil. Roast for 30 minutes, or until the vegetables are caramelized and any liquid has evaporated. Leave to cool.

TRANSFER the roasted veg to a food processor, add the remaining ingredients and pulse until roughly chopped. Form the mixture into 4 patties and chill for 1 hour.

HEAT a little oil in a large frying pan, add the patties and cook for about 15 minutes, turning occasionally, until piping hot all the way through.

SERVE the burgers in wholegrain buns with sliced tomatoes, grated cheese, avocado, rocket and Pink Pickled Onions with Lime & Bay.

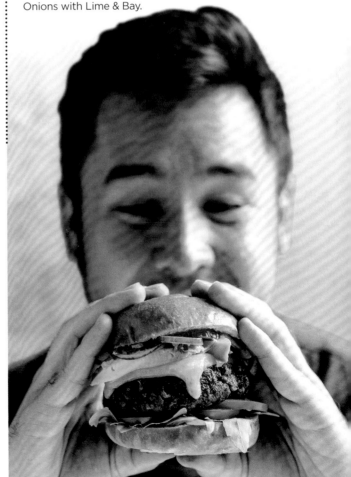

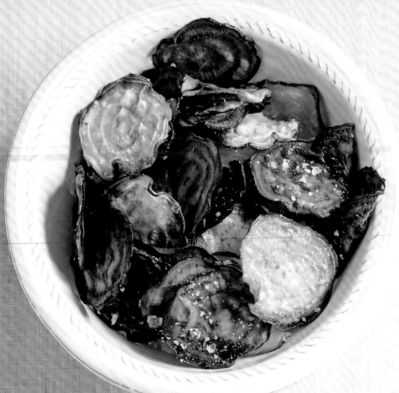

BEETROOT CRISPS

Crisp and light, these make an amazing alternative to tortillas for dipping into guacamole. Want to get fancier? Serve the same crisps topped with cubed avocado, chopped onion, lemon and chilli for rustic, healthy homemade canapés.

SERVES 2
PREP TIME 5 MINUTES
COOK TIME 10–12 MINUTES

······································

2 RAW WHOLE BEETROOTS
2 TBSP OLIVE OIL
1 TSP SALT

PREHEAT the oven to 180°C/Gas Mark 4.

SLICE the beetroots very finely using a mandoline, then transfer to 1–2 large baking sheets. Toss in the oil, then sprinkle with the salt.

BAKE for 10–12 minutes until crisp, then leave to cool.

SERVE when cooled or store the crisps in an airtight container for up to 2 weeks.

VARIATIONS

SPICY

Make the crisps as above, replacing the 1 tsp salt with 1 tsp **cayenne pepper** and ½ tsp **salt**. Bake as above.

SMOKY

Make the crisps as above, replacing the 1 tsp salt with 1 tsp **sweet smoked paprika** and ½ tsp **salt**. Bake as above.

SEA SALT & VINEGAR

Make the crisps as above, replacing the 1 tsp salt with ½ tsp **salt** and sprinkling with 1 tbsp **white wine vinegar**. Bake as above.

BEET & BLUEBERRY SMOOTHIE

Really hate the earthy flavour of beetroot? No problem! There are a few simple tricks to make it totally unnoticeable: adding acid, adding sweetness and serving it cold all effectively mask this flavour. The best way to combine all three tricks is to make a smoothie. Both the sweetness from the fruit and the acid in the lime help distract from the woodsy flavour, with ice lowering the temperature of the smoothie, which makes it harder for our bodies to perceive the earthiness.

SERVES 1

PREP TIME 5 MINUTES

....

1 COOKED BEETROOT, ROUGHLY CHOPPED

150ML CLOUDY APPLE JUICE

50G FRESH BLUEBERRIES

50G STRAWBERRIES, HULLED

FINELY GRATED ZEST AND JUICE OF 1 LIME

HANDFUL OF ICE

BLITZ all the ingredients together in a blender or food processor until smooth.

POUR into a glass and serve immediately.

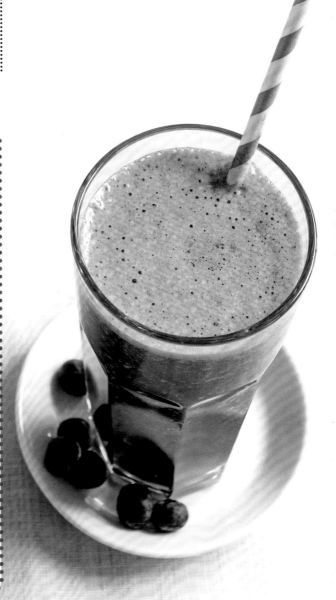

EAT THEIR GREENS

Beet leaves are not only edible, but also positively delicious. (The same is true of chard because the two crops are actually one and the same species.) They don't fare too shabbily in the nutrition stakes either. Like other dark green leafy veg, they are an excellent source of vitamins A, C and E and calcium, with 50 per cent more magnesium and potassium than even nutritional heavyweight kale. With five to six times more folate than the roots themselves, scoffing the greens that are often sold still attached to bunches of beetroot (rather than consigning them to the bin) will give you 'superfood' for free.

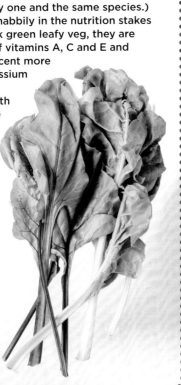

MUSHROOMS

Mushrooms are biologically more closely related to animals than they are to plants, belonging to a kingdom of their own – fungi – which may explain why they have a range of unique nutritional benefits when it comes to vegetables. They are rare non-animal sources of the essential nutrients selenium and vitamin D2, two of the most common deficiencies even in developed countries. Like plants they are also rich in fibre, including two specific types found in no other veg, chitin and lentinan, which emerging research suggests may have profound effects on immune function and blood pressure. Best of both worlds! Scientific research into the health benefits of mushrooms might be in its infancy but here's what the lab geeks have uncovered so far.

♡ VITAMIN D DYNAMITE

Vitamin D helps control the levels of minerals such as calcium and phosphorus in our bodies, which are essential for healthy bones and teeth. Low levels of it have been linked to poor immune function, clinical depression and even declines in mental function such as Alzheimer's disease. Although our bodies can amazingly manufacture their own vitamin D when our skin is exposed to sunlight, a huge number of people are still not getting enough of this essential nutrient, especially during the autumn and winter.

As it can be hard to consume sufficient vitamin D through our diets alone, government agencies, such as Public Health England, have even gone as far as recommending that *everyone* should consider taking a supplement, especially in the colder months. In the case of people with darker skin – such as people of South Asian or African descent – who may not be able to manufacture enough vitamin D even in summer, this advice extends year-round. What happens if you live in sunny Oz, instead of chilly Britain? Well, it seems like you still may be at risk, with 30 per cent of Australians deficient in the vitamin.

Fortunately, mushrooms – if treated correctly – can be an excellent source of vitamin D; in fact, the very best of all common foods per serving, with just three regular button mushrooms potentially providing your full recommended daily intake. Compare that to some of the other good dietary sources of vitamin D such as eggs (you'd have to eat up to 10 a day), tuna (1 entire can) or roast turkey breast (a whopping whole kilo) and mushrooms stack up pretty amazingly. One animal study has even shown that adding vitamin D-rich mushrooms to diets low in the nutrient could significantly improve learning and memory, and prevent the memory impairment associated with dementia – if you happen to be a lab mouse, that is, prompting the question of whether similar results could be found in humans. While correct processing is essential to unlocking the vitamin D potential in mushrooms, it is super-quick and easy for anyone to do (see page 90).

♡ IMMUNITY SUPPORT

Tuck into a generous serving of dried shiitake mushrooms a day – cooked whichever way you fancy – and what happens? Well, within 4 weeks you could see a doubling in your body's number of killer T-cells (the foot soldiers of your immune system that seek out and destroy infected cells), according to a clinical trial at the University of Florida. This boost in numbers was also accompanied by an improvement in their function, making them more responsive to the threat of infection.

This might sound great – after all, who wouldn't like a stronger immune system? – but in people with allergies and auto-immune disorders like rheumatoid arthritis, an overactive immune system can backfire, resulting in painful inflammatory symptoms that can ironically lead to an increased risk of cardiovascular diseases. What was so exciting about this study, therefore, was that the people eating the mushrooms actually showed lower levels of inflammation, suggesting eating shiitakes could boost immunity without the potential downsides.

Similar results were also found in a trial on plain old white button mushrooms, which showed a 50 per cent boost in Type A antibodies (the first line of immune defence in your gut) after just a week of eating a large daily serving. These levels even stayed elevated for a week after the subjects stopped consuming the mushrooms, before eventually dropping back to baseline. And all this without an increase in inflammation – a pretty great reward for scoffing a delicious, affordable, versatile, meaty-tasting veg.

Portobello mushrooms have **TWICE** the immune-boosting **chitin** of **button mushrooms**

🧺 BEST OF THE BEST

The wonderful thing about mushrooms is it appears you don't have to seek out the fancy exotic or wild types to reap the benefits. In fact, research suggests that button mushrooms are one of the best types, alongside the deliciously smoky shiitakes that are becoming increasingly common in supermarkets everywhere. Here is how they stack up in the nutritional stakes.

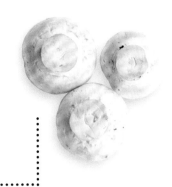

Button

Spanish researchers investigated eight different types of edible mushrooms and found that buttons had the second-highest levels of polyphenols – much higher than even posh chanterelles and twice those of exotic oysters. OK, so they did admittedly come sloppy seconds to porcini, which had almost double those of the button type. However, considering their far lower price and the realistic amount you are likely to eat in each dish (most recipes only call for tiny amounts of porcini), button mushrooms come out pretty darn well. Oh, and if you want to go one better, it appears that chestnut mushrooms, which are just a darker strain of white button mushrooms, may have even more polyphenols than their paler cousins, too.

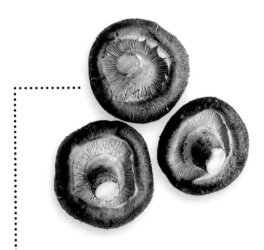

GO FOR THE BIG BOYS

Chitin is a complex carb that is thought may be at least partially responsible for the potential immune-boosting properties of mushrooms. In a study at the University of Illinois that analysed the nutritional composition of a range of mushrooms, researchers found that chitin levels were the highest in portobello mushrooms. Despite being only slightly more mature chestnut mushrooms that are harvested a few days later, portobellos contained more than twice the chitin gram for gram. Indeed, it seems across the board chitin concentrations increase as the mushroom grows, so always go for the big boys.

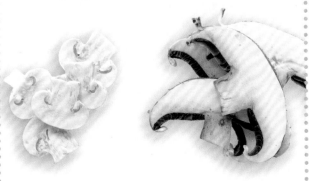

Shiitake

These tasty Asian mushrooms might have far fewer polyphenols than button types, but they more than make up for it in the fibre stakes, containing double that of the regular white sort. One of these fibres, lentinan, has attracted the attention of researchers for its impact on immune function in numerous animal and test-tube studies. With evidence across a number of small trials that it can improve survival rates of gastric cancer patients when administered in conjunction with chemotherapy, compared with chemo alone, it is even prescribed as part of conventional medicine in Japan. It might be the lentinan that is – at least in part – responsible for the impressive immune-boosting effect reported in the Florida University trial on page 88. Sadly, and frankly surprisingly, very few other good-quality clinical trials have been conducted, so it is very much a case of wait and see here.

I'd sidestep the overpriced runty ones sold alongside other dried mushrooms in regular supermarkets, though, and track them down in Asian food stores where they can sell for less than a quarter of the normal price.

SOLAR-POWERED NUTRITION

Doing one simple thing to your shop-bought fresh mushrooms can transform them from containing virtually zero vitamin D to one of nature's richest food sources in as little as an hour or two, according to Penn State University. Popped on a sunny windowsill, the mushrooms (which commercially are grown in near total darkness) will react to the UV light, churning out loads more of the antioxidant vitamin to defend themselves from damage from solar radiation.

The Penn State team found that a serving of white button mushrooms exposed to UV lamps for just *1 second* could go from containing essentially zero vitamin D, to an astonishing 824 per cent of your daily recommended intake. When they tried the same thing with shiitake and oyster mushrooms, their vitamin D content skyrocketed way over a thousand times what you need to consume each day. In the world of food science, this really is as close as you can get to alchemy.

With such tiny amounts of UV light needed to create such an enormous impact, it doesn't have to be a blazingly sunny day for you to do this at home either – simply lay your mushrooms out on a windowsill for an hour or two anytime between 10am and 3pm and their levels should peak significantly. As the gill tissue (the brown underside of the mushroom caps) is more sensitive to light, placing them with the gills facing up will trigger the strongest spike. You can now even buy special vitamin D-rich mushrooms at a premium price in some posher supermarkets where this UV treatment has already been done for you. Just three of these mushrooms should give you your entire daily dose. But as tumbling your mushrooms out on the work surface for an hour or so will do the exact same job, you may want to save your cash.

ROAST SHIITAKE WITH OLIVES & CARAMELIZED ONIONS

One of the richest sources of umami known to man, shiitakes are my go-to ingredient for adding a rich, comforting flavour to all sorts of dishes. But why not go one further? This recipe combines shiitakes with umami-rich soy and black olives and roasts them to concentrate the savoury trifecta. Delicious and versatile in salads, sandwiches, as a base for soups and pasta sauces or as a side dish on their own.

SERVES 2

PREP TIME 10 MINUTES, PLUS STANDING

COOK TIME 20 MINUTES

100G DRIED SHIITAKE MUSHROOMS

1 TBSP SOY SAUCE

1 TBSP SHERRY

300ML HOT CHICKEN OR VEGETABLE STOCK

50G PITTED BLACK OLIVES, SLICED

1 TBSP OLIVE OIL

1 GARLIC CLOVE, MINCED

1 ONION, SLICED

PREHEAT the oven to 220°C/Gas Mark 7.

PLACE the mushrooms, soy sauce, sherry and hot stock in a heatproof bowl and stir well to combine. Cover and leave the mushrooms to rehydrate for 10 minutes. Drain off any excess liquid, squeezing the mushrooms dry, then roughly slice the mushrooms.

SCATTER the mushrooms on a large baking sheet. Add the olives, oil, garlic and onion and toss with the mushrooms. Roast for 20 minutes, stirring halfway through the cooking time.

HOW TO SERVE

(1) SHIITAKE, MANDARIN & SPINACH SALAD

Toss together 1 x quantity **Roast Shiitake with Olives &
Caramelized Onions**, a small handful each of **mint** and **basil**
leaves, 200g **mandarin slices**, 200g sliced **cherry tomatoes**,
2 large handfuls of **spinach** and 50g **pine nuts** in a serving
bowl. Drizzle over 1 tbsp **olive oil** and 1 tsp **balsamic vinegar**
and serve.

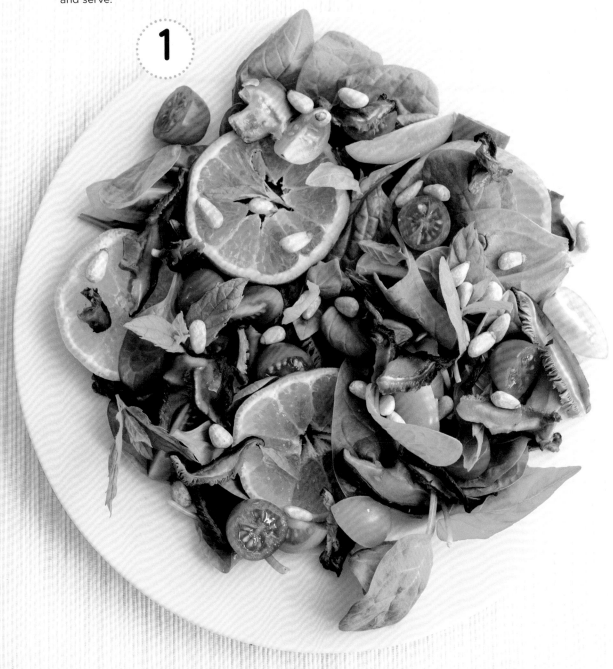

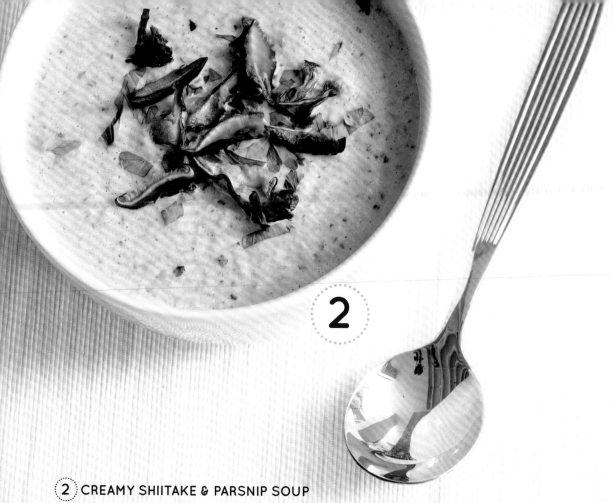

② CREAMY SHIITAKE & PARSNIP SOUP

Setting a little of the mixture aside for garnish, place 1 x quantity **Roast Shiitake with Olives & Carmelized Onions**, 1 grated **parsnip**, 1 litre **milk**, 150ml **white wine**, 50g **flaked almonds** and 150ml **beef or vegetable stock** in a saucepan and simmer gently for 15 minutes until the parsnip is tender. Transfer the soup to a blender or food processor and blitz until smooth. Reheat if necessary, then ladle into bowls, drizzle with **double cream**, and garnish with the reserved **Roast Shiitake with Olives & Carmelized Onions** and chopped **parsley**.

COOK THEM HOWEVER YOU LIKE

The great news is both drying and cooking seem to have very little impact on the vitamin D or immune-boosting fibres in mushrooms, meaning you can feel free to eat them however you want.

If you are stuck for ideas, however, there is plenty of inspiration here to get you started, all using the same super-versatile base recipe for Roast Shiitake with Olives & Caramelized Onions on page 90.

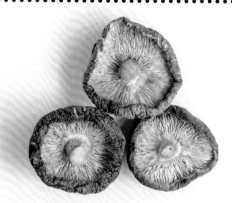

(3) SHIITAKE NO-MEATBALLS

Blitz 1 x quantity **Roast Shiitake with Olives & Carmelized Onions**, 200g drained and rinsed canned **black beans**, 2 slices of **wholemeal bread**, torn into chunks, 1 tsp **smoked paprika**, 1 tsp **dried oregano**, 1 tsp **dried garlic** and 1 tsp grated **Parmesan cheese** in a food processor. Shape the mixture into balls and space evenly on a baking sheet. Drizzle with 1 tbsp **olive oil** and roast in a preheated oven, 200°C/Gas Mark 6, for 20 minutes. Serve with **Roasted Cherry Tomato Sauce** (see page 25) in 4 **wholemeal sub rolls** with **mozzarella cheese** and a bunch of **watercress**. These balls are also pretty spectacular atop spaghetti, simmered in creamy curries or paired with old-school mash, gravy and sautéed greens. Yum.

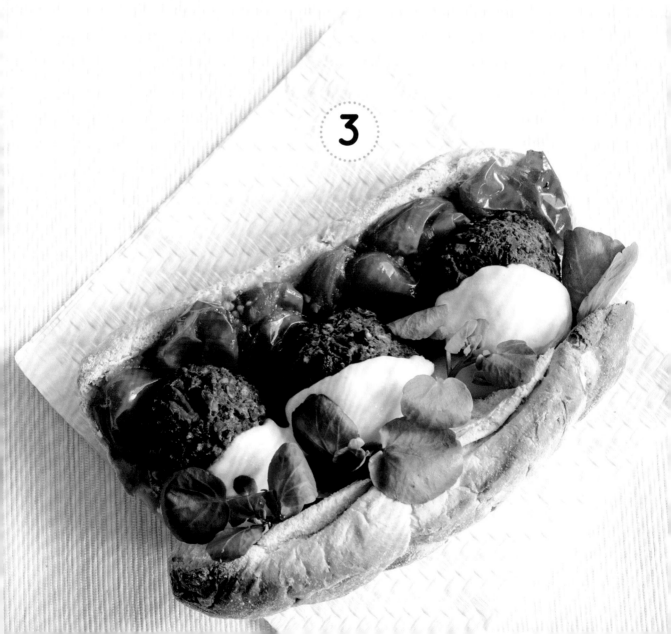

CARROTS

With over three times your daily dose of vitamin A per 100g serving, along with a ton of healthy fibre, and all wrapped in a sweet-tasting, brightly coloured veg that looks great on your plate, it's no wonder carrots are one of the world's most popular veg. With some simple tips to select, store and cook, you can make them even better. Here goes...

♡ EYE HEALTH

Right in the centre of your retina there is a yellow spot filled with orange pigments called carotenes. Some (but not all) studies point to the ability of two carotenes here called lutein and zeaxanthin to protect the retina from damage caused by UV light, improving visual acuity and reducing the risk of cataracts and age-related macular degeneration – the leading cause of blindness in the over 65s in the developed world. Where do we get these carotenes from? Well, carrots are an excellent source. Yet the average US diet contains just 1–3mg a day, far less than the 6mg amount believed to confer a protective effect. Enjoy more carrots in exchange for potentially reducing your risk of vision loss? It seems like a fair deal to me.

♡ REDUCED CANCER RISK?

One Japanese study that followed over 15,000 older men for 20 years found that while general fruit and veg consumption appeared to have little effect on the risk of developing prostate cancer, intake of one form of carotene called alpha-carotene was associated with close to a 50 per cent lower incidence of the disease. Similar results were also found in a much larger US study that followed 120,000 men and women to track the association between carotene intake and lung cancer. While other carotenes had little effect, alpha-carotene intake was linked to a far lower incidence. For a single nutrient, this is pretty huge.

Aside from canned pumpkin (when was the last time you ate that?), the highest commonly available source of alpha-carotene is – you guessed it – cooked carrots. Considering the very modest amounts associated with a reduced risk (as little as the equivalent of munching on two cooked carrots a week in the Japanese study), this is a habit that is easy to adopt for most people and is just another reason to eat more carrots.

EAT THEM YOUNG WITH THE SKIN ON

According to the *Journal of Food, Agriculture and Environment*, the polyphenols in carrots are not distributed evenly throughout the veg, but concentrated in their outer layers, particularly in the skin. In fact, the simple act of peeling carrots could more than halve their polyphenol levels instantly. Sacrilege! As younger carrots contain proportionately far more skin and less core, owing to their thinner size, trendy baby veg just might be a better option, especially as, unlike regular-sized carrots, these are usually served unpeeled. One study published in the *Canadian Journal of Plant Science* supports this idea, observing that the high level of polyphenols in young carrot roots falls continuously during the first 3 months until harvest. Prefer baby veg? Well, here is your perfect excuse.

TREAT 'EM MEAN, KEEP 'EM KEEN

OK, so here is a weird one from Texas A&M University for those who prefer their carrots raw. Cutting fresh carrots and letting them sit in the fridge can trigger them to generate significantly more polyphenols. The more damage you inflict (i.e. the finer you cut them) the more the still-living carrot tissue reacts by trying to protect itself, sending the levels of these beneficial compounds soaring. Shred on a grater, bung them in the fridge and the same carrots could have roughly two and a half times the polyphenols and a whopping 12-fold more antioxidant activity just days later. While all this planning ahead might sound like a lot of faff, it does have one important potential benefit for lazy cooks like me. It suggests that shop-bought carrot batons, or better yet, grated carrot salad may well have more of the good stuff than homemade.

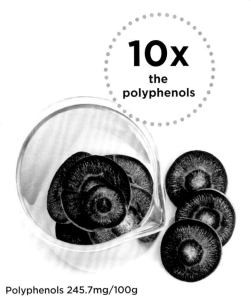

10x
the
polyphenols

Polyphenols 245.7mg/100g

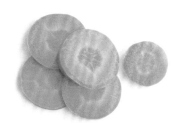

Polyphenols 31.0mg/100g

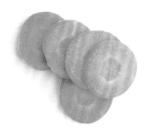

Polyphenols 29.3mg/100g

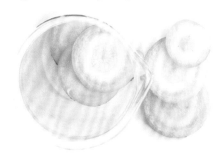

Polyphenols 21.5mg/100g

HIGHEST POLYPHENOLS

LOWEST POLYPHENOLS

Purple

Purple carrots predate the development of today's new-fangled orange varieties by hundreds of years. Their deep purple hue comes from the same group of anthocyanin compounds that give blueberries and red wine their potential health benefits. Yet don't let this fool you into thinking they lack carotenes. In fact, they contain well over twice the levels of these orange pigments according to the University of Lincolnshire; their presence is just masked by the purple ones. Combine a double whammy of these carotenes and anthocyanins and what do you get? Carrots with on average an astonishing ten times more polyphenols than roots of other colours, according the University of Krakow in Poland. They might still be the preserve of farmers' markets and independent greengrocers, where they sell for a little more than regular ones (10 per cent more in my local store), but slowly the word is getting out. The more purple your carrot, the better. So if given the choice, for the very highest polyphenol content pick varieties that are maroon to the core, rather than the orange ones with purple skins.

....

Red

Red carrots are a group of varieties common in East Asia that have a slightly higher carotene content than the standard orange ones, including lycopene, which gives tomatoes and watermelons their red colour (see page 22). These do come with added benefits but nowhere near the scale of purple ones.

....

Orange

The familiar orange carrot is the result of a random mutation that was first noticed in Holland 300-odd years ago. Despite the fact that they contained significantly less phytonutrients than the older purple form, these were popularized by the Dutch royal family (a dynastic order known as 'The House of Orange') who then spread them across the world. They are still an excellent source of nutrition compared to the other non-purple varieties, and, of course, far more commonly available, so pick them over their paler cousins every time.

....

Yellow & white

Yellow carrots are really just orange ones with even less carotene. White ones are essentially devoid of pretty much all of it, meaning these pale contenders offer up as little as half the polyphenols of the regular orange carrot, while simultaneously being more expensive and harder to track down. Why do it to yourself?

GLAZED YOUNG CARROTS WITH BEETROOT STEMS

Want to triple the betacarotene in your carrots? Just cook them. A University of California study found that female subjects consuming cooked carrots absorbed three times more betacarotene than when they ate the exact same amount of the substance in raw carrots.

By braising carrots in their own juices this recipe prevents the potential loss of up to 20 per cent of the carotenes, 25 per cent of the sugars and a large chunk of the vitamin C that can occur in the traditional boiling method, where so much of the good stuff is lost to the cooking water. Teaming up a mix of orange, red and purple carrots with the tender stems of beets makes this a stunning veggie course that's as tasty as it is healthy.

SERVES 4 AS A SIDE DISH

PREP TIME 15 MINUTES

COOK TIME 15–20 MINUTES

....

500G CARROTS (AIM FOR MIXED COLOURS AND UNIFORM SIZES)

FINELY GRATED ZEST AND JUICE OF 1 MANDARIN

1 TBSP HONEY

1 TBSP BUTTER

1 GARLIC CLOVE, FINELY CHOPPED

STALKS AND LEAVES FROM 1 BUNCH OF BEETROOTS, LARGER STALKS ROUGHLY CHOPPED

1 TBSP CHOPPED PARSLEY, OR A FEW CARROT LEAVES (WHICH ARE RELATED TO PARSLEY)

SALT AND PEPPER

PACK the carrots into a large, shallow saucepan, add the mandarin zest and juice, honey, butter and garlic, then season with a little salt and pepper. Cover and cook over a medium-low heat for 10–15 minutes.

ADD the beetroot stalks and leaves. Re-cover and cook for another 5 minutes until the carrots are tender.

SPRINKLE over the parsley or carrot leaves and serve.

DON'T FEAR THE FAT

Want to up carotene levels even more? Well, a good glug of olive oil has been found to increase the bioavailability of cooked carrots according to a Spanish research team, boosting it by as much as 50 per cent. This is because carotenes are fat soluble, so oil serves as the perfect vehicle to draw them out of the carrots into a form that is easier for your body to get at. Similar results have been found for tomatoes (see page 26), winter squash and leafy greens, and pretty much any veg that contains carotenes.

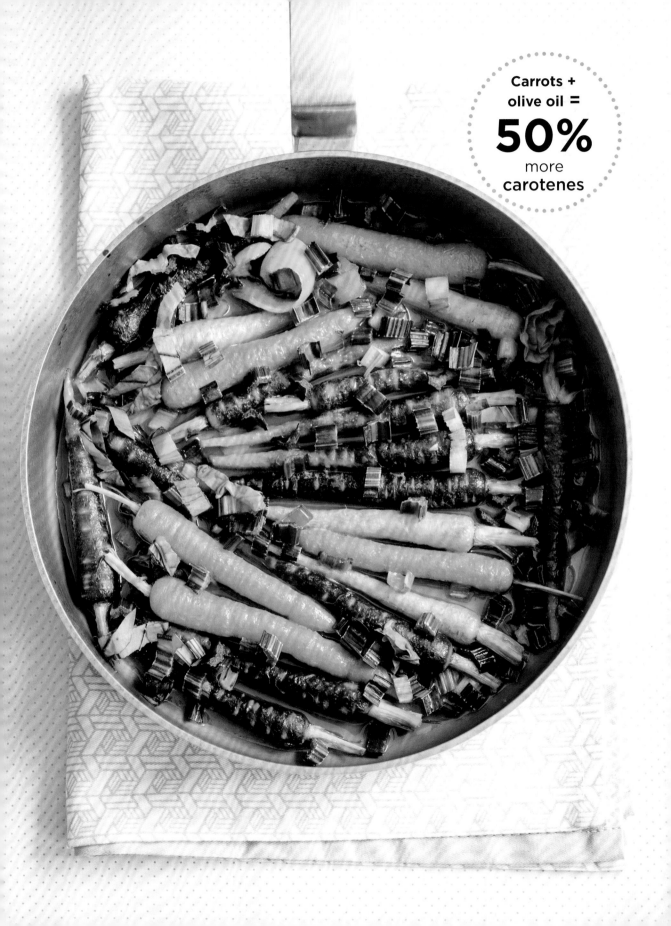

Carrots +
olive oil =
50%
more
carotenes

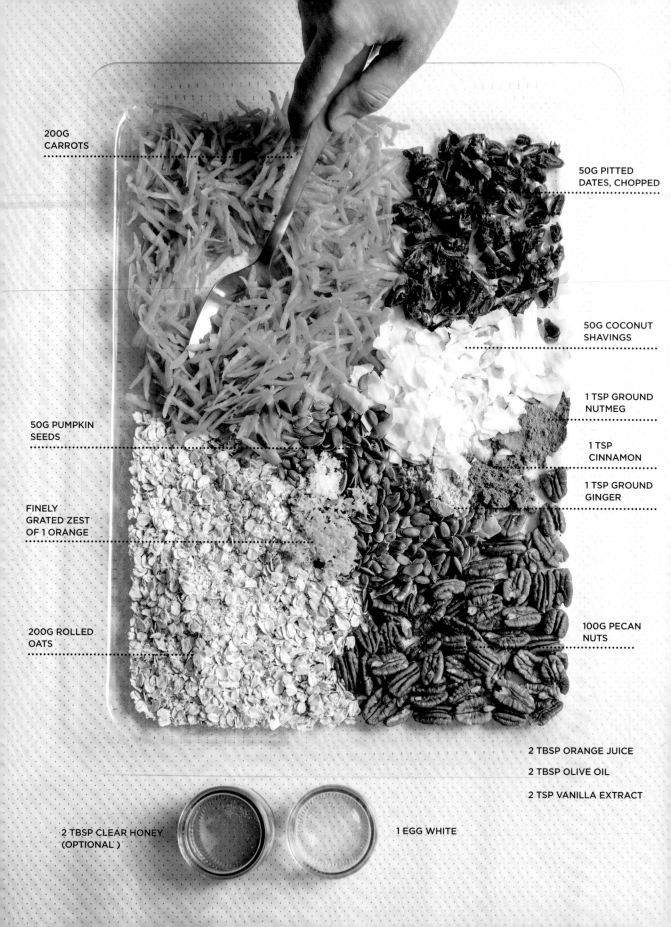

200G
CARROTS

50G PITTED
DATES, CHOPPED

50G COCONUT
SHAVINGS

1 TSP GROUND
NUTMEG

1 TSP
CINNAMON

1 TSP GROUND
GINGER

50G PUMPKIN
SEEDS

FINELY
GRATED ZEST
OF 1 ORANGE

100G PECAN
NUTS

200G ROLLED
OATS

2 TBSP ORANGE JUICE

2 TBSP OLIVE OIL

2 TSP VANILLA EXTRACT

2 TBSP CLEAR HONEY
(OPTIONAL)

1 EGG WHITE

CARROT CAKE GRANOLA

The sweet flavour and beautiful colour of carrots make them a super-versatile way to sneak extra veg into all sorts of meals as a replacement for carbs – even at breakfast. This simple granola ditches the sky-high added-sugar content of many traditional recipes in favour of loads of fruit, veg and nuts – which make up 60 per cent of each serving.

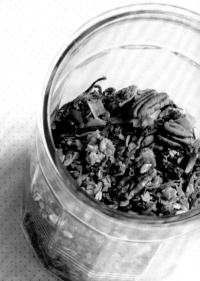

MAKES 500G
PREP TIME 15 MINUTES, PLUS COOLING
COOK TIME 45 MINUTES

PREHEAT the oven to 180°C/Gas Mark 4.

GRATE the carrots on the thickest setting of your grater, then squeeze out the excess juice. Sprinkle the orange juice over the shavings (this will help retain their colour) and toss to combine.

SPREAD out the carrot gratings in a large baking tin and bake for 15 minutes. Remove from the oven and leave to cool for 10 minutes, leaving the oven on.

ADD all the remaining ingredients to the cooled carrots and toss together to combine the mix into a moist rubble.

RETURN to the oven and bake for another 30 minutes. Mix halfway through baking to ensure even cooking. The granola will crisp up on cooling. Store in an airtight container.

DITCH THE MILK

Instead of having a massive bowl of granola with milk, which makes it instantly soggy (why does anyone do that, anyway?), I like to serve just a few tablespoons as a crunchy sprinkle on a bowl of fruit and protein-packed Greek yogurt. A simple way to up the fruit and veg content even further while slashing calories almost in half.

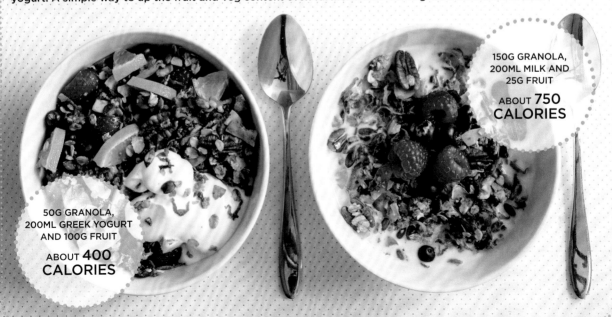

150G GRANOLA, 200ML MILK AND 25G FRUIT

ABOUT **750** CALORIES

50G GRANOLA, 200ML GREEK YOGURT AND 100G FRUIT

ABOUT **400** CALORIES

WINTER SQUASHES

Who cares about the onset of winter when you can have the sticky, golden, deliciousness these guys offer up? Packed with antioxidant carotenes, vitamin A and a good source of vitamin C, they are as nutritious as they are tasty – sharing many of the health benefits of carrots (see page 94). Here's a few tips and tricks to get even more goodness out of them.

TAKE YOUR TIME

Fresh food in season is always better, right? Well, not in the case of squashes. In fact, they noticeably increase their sugar content after a month of storage at 10°C. These sugars are used to fuel the creation of carotenes, improving both their colour and potential nutrition. It's these carotenes that are then broken down to create the aroma compounds that give winter squashes their characteristic buttery, caramel aroma. Sweeter, healthier, more flavoursome squash in exchange for little more than patience. A win-win all round, really! Butternut squashes require a bit longer, peaking in sugar and carotenes after 2 months, at which point their levels of carotenes can shoot up as much as 50 per cent.

If we simply stopped calling squashes an autumn veg and started viewing them as a winter one, we would give them an extra couple of months to start generating better flavour and nutrition. Wait until winter to buy them or pop autumn-bought ones in a cool place like a garage, give them a couple of weeks and enjoy their added benefits.

CAROTENES ARE SKIN DEEP

As with most fruit and veg, the skin of winter squashes contains far more protective nutrients, such as antioxidant carotenes, than the flesh. With many times more carotenes than the rest of the fruit in most varieties, the skin often has a sweet flavour all of its own, so simply not bothering to peel squashes will up their flavour, too. In some varieties, especially the classic 'Jack-o'-lantern' types, there can be an astonishing 27 times more carotenes in their bright orange skins than in their pale flesh. This difference is so great that by simply eating the slices with skin and all you can get a fivefold increase in carotenes per serving than if you just scooped up the flesh.

OVENS UP THE NUTRITION

Cooking is essential to bring out the fullest, caramel flavour of winter squashes, and by excellent coincidence research has shown that the same process can cause their nutrient content to soar. Malaysian researchers found that the betacarotene content of winter squashes can quadruple after just a few minutes of heat, with the lycopene (see page 22) content rocketing up an amazing 40 times.

But the exact method of cooking can make an important difference, too. Because many of the nutrients in winter squash can leach out into the cooking water, I would skip boiling (or steaming) and go for baking or roasting instead. The United States Department of Agriculture found that this simple swap could give you 50 per cent more vitamins A and C. Sorry, microwave ovens don't count. In fact, one study reported that just a few minutes of zapping could knock the carotene content of butternut squash by 30 per cent.

Get

5X

the carotenes by not bothering to peel the squash

HOKKAIDO
Carotenes
70mg/kg

CROWN PRINCE
Carotenes
65mg/kg

MUSCAT DE
PROVENCE
Carotenes
47mg/kg

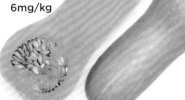

BUTTERNUT
Carotenes
6mg/kg

ACORN
Carotenes
2mg/kg

BABY BEAR
Carotenes
2mg/kg

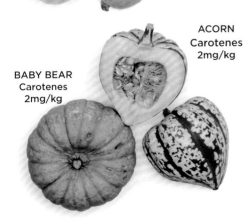

HIGHEST CAROTENES

LOWEST CAROTENES

True winter squashes

Most squashes belong to a species called *Cucurbita maxima*, which are all far higher in sugars, aroma chemicals and carotenes than butternut, Jack-o'-lantern and decorative squashes, making them both tastier and more nutritious! With nearly 12 times the carotenes of boring old butternut, Hokkaido is the 'Big Daddy' of squash nutrition according to a German research team. Other great examples include Crown Prince, Hubbard and Bon Bon. A single 100g serving of pretty much any member of this bright orange, intensely sweet species contains more than twice your recommended daily intake of vitamin A. The dense, creamy flesh even contains 50 per cent more fibre than butternut squash (and three times the fibre of soggy old Jack-o'-lantern-type pumpkins), so it's amazing that these aren't more commonly eaten.

Butternut squash

This is the darling of supermarkets because of its small size (perfect for small families) and ridiculously long shelf life. Belonging to a different species, *Curcubita moschata*, butternut squash has only a third the vitamin A of squash like Hubbard and Hokkaido and more than 80 per cent fewer carotenes, it is also notoriously watery in texture, with far less sugar and aroma chemicals. If you want to make profit of your supermarket balance sheet, this one's for you; if you are looking for flavour or nutrition, give it a wide berth.

There is one exception however to this general rule for this species, a quirky round variety of butternut called Muscat de Provence that is uncharacteristically high in carotenes, containing almost 70 per cent as much as Hokkaido according to the German study. Despite its impressive antioxidant payload, it still lacks the sweetness and dense flesh of the real deal. Amazing colour, not such amazing flavour.

Jack-o'-lantern & decorative squashes

With many fewer carotenes than even the lowly butternut, these guys aren't really good for much else. Closely related to courgettes and marrows, they belong to a third species called *Curcubuta pepo*, which lacks the high sugar content and rich aromatics that create that classic caramelized, 'pumpkin' flavour.

One of the worst offenders is the beautiful acorn squash that adorns the window displays of fancy supermarkets each autumn, which has a shocking 95 per cent less vitamin A than Hokkaido. You would have to eat literally 20 servings of its soggy, insipid flesh to get the carotene benefit of just one of the tastiest Hokkaido squashes as noted above. I know which one I would pick. Loads of style here, but sadly very little substance.

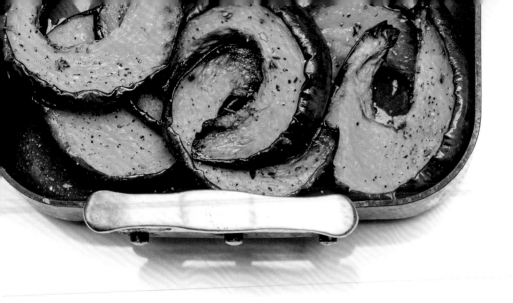

EASY ROAST WINTER SQUASH

Crisp on the outside, gooey in the middle, this is the healthiest and simplest possible way to cook winter squash. No peeling, just knock-out pure squash flavour for very little effort. When roast winter squash is blitzed up to a smooth, golden puree it can be used as a replacement for milk or water in pretty much any recipe – from soups and curries to pancakes. A sneaky way to significantly up flavour and nutrition with leftover veg.

SERVES 4 AS A SIDE DISH

PREP TIME 5 MINUTES

COOK TIME 45 MINUTES

....

600G WINTER SQUASH, SLICED AND DESEEDED

OLIVE OIL, FOR DRIZZLING

1 TBSP HONEY

SALT

PREHEAT the oven to 200°C/Gas Mark 6.

ARRANGE the squash slices on a baking sheet, drizzle with olive oil and the honey and sprinkle with salt. Roast for 45 minutes until soft.

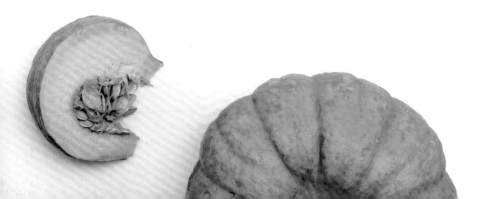

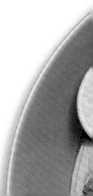

WINTER SQUASH & COCONUT LAKSA

Smooth, sweet winter squash enriches this comforting Southeast Asian soup with loads more flavour and nutrition. Who knew squash and coconut were a foodie match made in heaven?

SERVES 4

PREP TIME 20 MINUTES

COOK TIME 10 MINUTES

••••••••••••••••••••••••••••••••

2 GARLIC CLOVES, MINCED

1 THUMB-SIZED PIECE OF FRESH ROOT GINGER, PEELED AND SLICED INTO MATCHSTICKS

4 TBSP LAKSA PASTE (RED THAI CURRY PASTE WILL DO AT A PUSH)

1 X 400ML CAN COCONUT MILK

2 TSBP FISH SAUCE

500G EASY ROAST WINTER SQUASH (SEE PAGE 102), BLITZED TO A SMOOTH PURÉE

200G RAW PEELED KING PRAWNS

TO SERVE

250G COOKED EGG NOODLES

4 SPRING ONIONS, SLICED

2 RED THAI CHILLIES, SLICED

4 MINT SPRIGS, LEAVES TORN FROM STEMS AND FINELY CHOPPED

2 TBSP POMEGRANATE SEEDS

300G HALVED AND COOKED TENDERSTEM BROCCOLI

LIME WEDGES

COMBINE all the ingredients, except for the prawns, in a large saucepan. Bring to the boil and simmer for 5 minutes.

ADD the prawns and cook for 2 minutes until they turn pink and are cooked through.

DIVIDE the noodles among 4 bowls, ladle over the soup and sprinkle over the spring onions, chillies, mint, pomegranate seeds and broccoli. Serve with lime wedges for squeezing over.

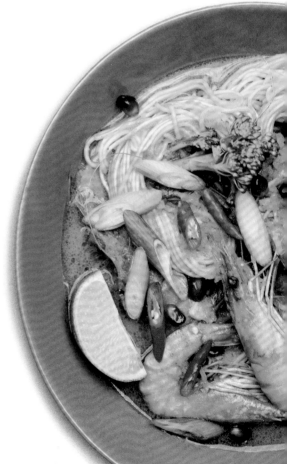

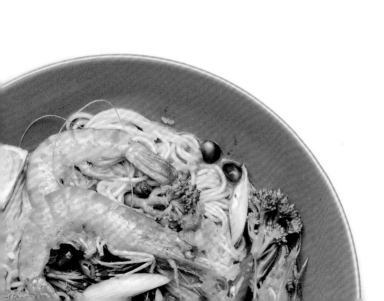

PUMPKIN & CORNMEAL HOECAKES

Puréed roast squash works its magic here too, giving this soul-food favourite a richer, more caramelized flavour and a healthy 25 per cent dose of extra veg to boot. As easy to make as they are indulgent, these hoecakes work well with any topping, savoury or sweet.

MAKES 10–12 HOECAKES

PREP TIME 15 MINUTES, PLUS STANDING

COOK TIME 15 MINUTES

200G ROAST PUMPKIN (SEE PAGE 102 FOR HOW TO ROAST WINTER SQUASH)

250G POLENTA OR CORNMEAL

3 EGGS

LARGE PINCH OF SALT

1 TSP MIXED SPICE

3 TBSP MELTED BUTTER, PLUS EXTRA FOR FRYING

FINELY GRATED ZEST OF 1 LEMON

2 TBSP GRANULATED STEVIA (BAKING BLEND)

100G PLAIN FLOUR

1 TSP BAKING POWDER

100ML MILK

BLITZ together the pumpkin, polenta, eggs, salt, mixed spice, melted butter, lemon zest and stevia in a food processor. Leave to stand for 5–10 minutes to let the polenta rehydrate.

ADD the flour, baking powder and milk and blitz again to make a batter.

HEAT 1 tsp butter in a large frying pan, then drop 2 tbsp of the mixture per hoecake into the pan, making sure they are well spaced apart. Cook over a medium heat for 2–3 minutes on each side until cooked through. Remove from the pan and keep warm in a low oven until all the hoecakes are made.

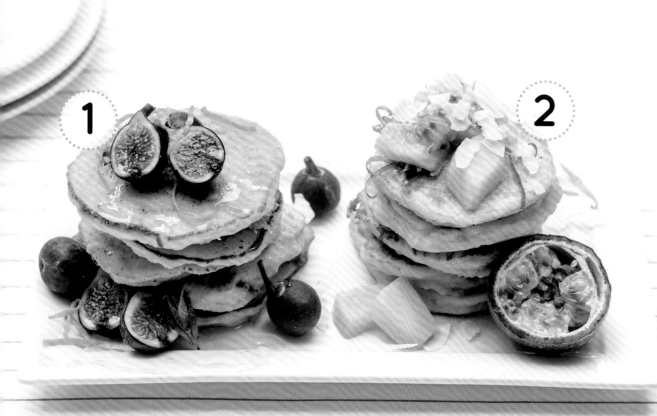

VARIATIONS

1

MED STYLE

Make the batter as opposite, omitting the stevia. Fold 50g grated **halloumi** and 4 chopped **fresh figs** into the batter before frying. Serve with sliced **figs**, **orange blossom honey**, finely grated **orange** zest and a few **mint** leaves.

2

THAI STYLE

Make the batter as opposite, folding in 50g **desiccated coconut** and the finely grated zest of ½ **lime** before frying. Serve with chopped **mango**, **passionfruit pulp**, **shredded coconut** and extra finely grated **lime** zest.

3

MEXICAN STYLE

Make the batter as opposite, omitting the stevia. Fold 50g grated **mild cheese** and 50g **sweetcorn** into the batter before frying. Top each serving with sliced **avocado**, **red chilli** slivers, and a little extra grated **mild cheese**.

4

AMERICAN STYLE

Make the batter as opposite, folding in 50g chopped **pecan nuts** before frying. Serve with sliced **banana**, **blueberries**, extra **pecan nuts** and **maple syrup**.

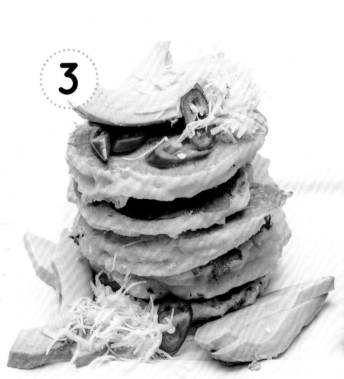

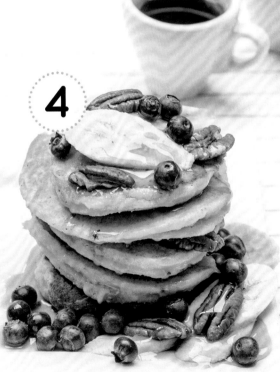

BANANAS

Bananas are officially the world's most commonly consumed fruit. Being essentially a block of satisfying starch and tasty sugar, this isn't that surprising. But sadly, in the vitamin, mineral and phytonutrient stakes, bananas rank pretty low when compared to other fruit and veg, especially when you match them calorie for calorie (they are, after all, packed with energy). While they might be a great source of vitamin B6 and contain a little vitamin C, even as a commonly cited source of potassium they contain half that of potatoes, beans and spinach. So why cover them in this book if they are just a slab of carbs? Well, it is the *type* of carbs that count.

♡ PREBIOTIC PROPERTIES

Bananas are rich in a special group of carbohydrates called 'resistant starches'. Our bodies aren't really able to break these down to access the calories they contain, meaning they 'resist' the digestion process.

Why is this a good thing? Well, first, despite filling us up more than regular starches, they theoretically contain zero calories. So far, so good. Secondly, being essentially indigestible to humans means these carbs pass straight through our bodies, acting more like fibre, slowing the impact of the carbs that *are* digestible on our blood sugar and, of course, keeping us regular. Thirdly, the one thing that *can* feast on resistant starches are friendly bacteria in your colon. A range of recent studies has linked gut microbe imbalances with everything from a higher risk of bowel cancer to depression and anxiety, obesity and impaired immune function. One of the best ways to keep the good guys in your guts in tiptop condition is to feed them with a regular supply of resistant starch – what science geeks call a 'prebiotic'.

Clinical trials have even shown that eating bananas can dramatically reduce the incidence of potentially life-threatening imbalances that cause severe diarrhoea in children, helping them come off intravenous drips and quelling bouts of vomiting faster than control groups. A large part of their efficacy is believed to be not the resistant starch itself, but a group of anti-inflammatory chemicals called short-chain fatty acids produced by the gut bacteria that eat these indigestible carbs.

These acids help maintain a healthy gut lining and stimulate the absorption of water and essential salts in the colon and from there even travel round the body to quell inflammation. For this very reason, bananas are a key part of the BRAT diet (Banana, Rice, Apple, Tea) that is a commonly recommended part of conventional treatment for patients with diarrhoea. A pretty perfect food for all-round gut health it seems.

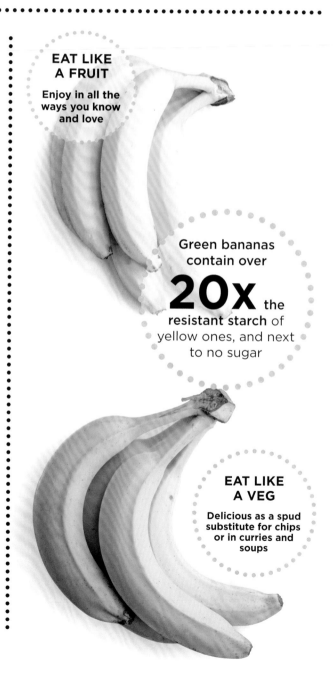

EAT LIKE A FRUIT

Enjoy in all the ways you know and love

Green bananas contain over

20x the **resistant starch** of yellow ones, and next to no sugar

EAT LIKE A VEG

Delicious as a spud substitute for chips or in curries and soups

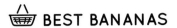 BEST BANANAS

Unless you live in the tropics or shop in some pretty fancy supermarkets, chances are every banana you have ever eaten comes from a single variety, the Dwarf Cavendish. Originally grown in the great glasshouses of the sixth Duke of Devonshire in his mansion at Chatsworth House in the 19th century, it was spread around the world through a network of imperial trading routes and now dominates international trade. However, despite virtually zero variety choice in most supermarkets, there is a type of banana that contains many times more resistant starch than others, not to mention way less sugar. Let me explain....

Go for green

The high sugar levels of the sweet yellow bananas we all know and love are generated during the process of ripening from the breakdown of resistant starch. So unripe, green bananas of the exact same variety contain bag-loads more of the good stuff, perhaps more than any other commonly eaten food....Wait, who on earth eats green bananas? Well, millions of people around the world do – from Latin America and the Caribbean to large parts of Asia and Africa – cooking and eating them not as a sweet fruit, but as a starchy vegetable that tastes much like a potato but with a richer, nuttier flavour.

To the uninitiated, this may seem a bit weird, but they make a delicious substitute for spuds or other starchy root veg, and have fewer calories and less impact on blood sugar, plus a hefty dose of prebiotic resistant starch. For the GI geeks (Glycaemic Index, see page 46), they are about as low as carbs go – ranking at about 30, they have a similar level to beans – keeping you fuller for far longer.

WHAT ABOUT PLANTAINS?

You may have noticed I have kept very quiet about plantains. These are a larger, starchier species of banana popularly sold in Asian and Afro-Caribbean grocery stores. It turns out that green plantains have a form of starch that is even more resistant than that found in regular bananas, which make them an even better source of prebiotics.

However, as plantains can be harder to hunt down, I have focused on the commonest type. If you are lucky enough to have the more exotic type at your local shop, by all means pick them every time.

THE FRUIT OF HAPPINESS?

Bananas are a rich natural source of serotonin, a human brain chemical associated with feelings of happiness and well-being. There's enough in them to significantly boost the levels in your blood too. The only problem? Serotonin cannot cross the blood–brain barrier, meaning it never gets to where it needs to go for it to work, no matter how many bananas you eat.

COOKING GREEN BANANAS

To be very honest, almost all starches are technically 'resistant' in their raw form, which is why no one really eats raw flour, rice or potatoes. You have to apply heat to them to soften the indigestible raw starches, turning them into the gel-like, calorie-dense deliciousness that our bodies can use. Believe me, I have read about (and tried) many ways to up my resistant starch intake by eating some of these carbs raw, and frankly, they are all horrendously unappetizing. From the chalky texture to their monotonously bland flavour, they are often quite literally hard to swallow.

But what makes green bananas so interesting is that they contain an unusual form of resistant starch that is not degraded but actually increased by heating, meaning they are still a great source of this starch even when cooked. Researchers have boiled them, fried them and even made them into bread and pasta, without unduly affecting their impact on blood sugar. In fact, in one study published in the *International Food Research Journal*, researchers found that cooking green bananas could double their resistant starch content.

A number of studies have found that chilling cooked bananas in a fridge could further increase their resistant starch by an extra 50 per cent, giving them almost three times the levels found in the raw stuff. Moral of the story? Cooked green bananas are one of the healthiest, tastiest carb sources going. Their leftovers, though, might be even better. See pages 109–110 for some recipe ideas to get you started.

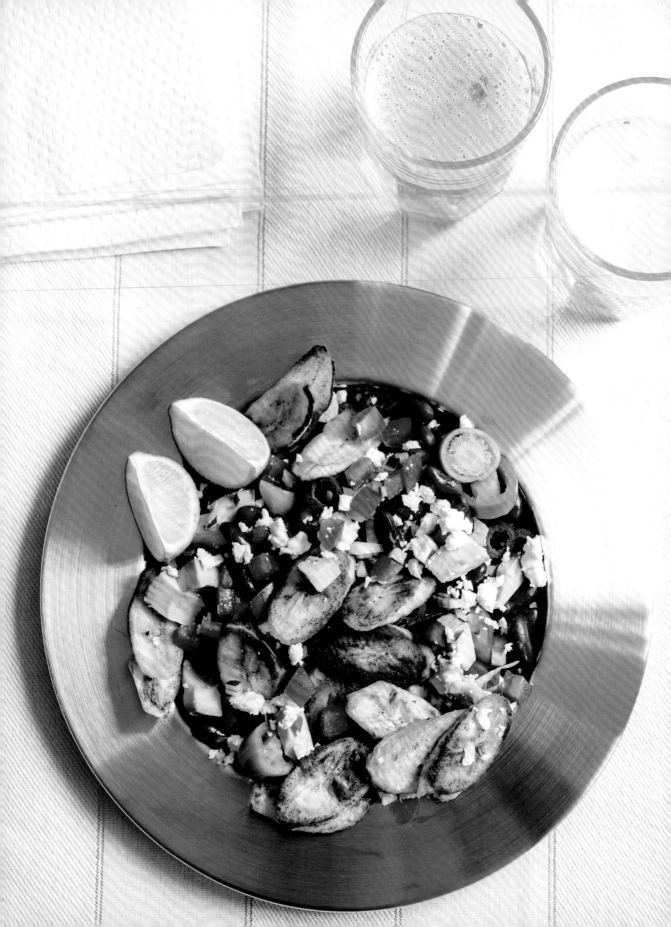

ECUADORIAN GREEN BANANA NACHOS

Yes, I know nachos aren't Ecuadorian but a 20th-century Tex-Mex concoction. Yet this is exactly how they often come served in the bars in downtown Quito, where I lived in my 20s, and where green banana chips are as common as the spud type.

SERVES 4
PREP TIME 15 MINUTES
COOK TIME 20 MINUTES

....

4 GREEN BANANAS

2 TBSP OLIVE OIL

1 TSP TURMERIC

½ TSP SALT

¼ TSP BLACK PEPPER

100G JALAPEÑO PEPPERS FROM A JAR

½ RED ONION, VERY FINELY DICED

1 LARGE TOMATO, DICED

1 LARGE AVOCADO, STONED, PEELED AND CUBED

200G DRAINED AND RINSED CANNED KIDNEY BEANS

50G PITTED BLACK OLIVES, SLICED

50G FETA CHEESE, CRUMBLED

LIME WEDGES, TO SERVE

PREHEAT the oven to 220°C/Gas Mark 7 and line a large baking sheet with nonstick baking paper.

PEEL the green bananas with a sharp knife (this isn't as easy as it is with ripe ones) and slice into pieces about 5mm thick.

PLACE the bananas in a bowl and toss together with the oil, turmeric, salt and pepper until the bananas are evenly coated.

SPREAD the slices over the prepared baking sheet in a single layer and bake for 20 minutes, or until golden brown, turning halfway through the cooking time.

ARRANGE the banana chips on a large serving platter, then top with the remaining ingredients. Serve with lime wedges for squeezing over.

SINGAPORE GREEN BANANA CURRY

This is my shamelessly Westernized take on my favourite curry, which they used to serve on Tuesdays at my school canteen in Singapore. Warming and creamy, this is comfort food, Southeast Asian style.

SERVES 4
PREP TIME 10 MINUTES
COOK TIME 15 MINUTES

....

4 GREEN BANANAS,
1 TBSP OLIVE OIL
1 ONION, FINELY SLICED
3 TBSP RED CURRY PASTE
1 TSP TURMERIC
400ML COCONUT MILK
1 RED PEPPER, CORED, DESEEDED AND SLICED
100G GREEN BEANS, TRIMMED AND SLICED INTO 2.5CM PIECES
1 GARLIC CLOVE, MINCED
1 TSP PEELED AND MINCED FRESH ROOT GINGER
SALT AND PEPPER

TO SERVE
3 RED CHILLIES, SLICED
25G CORIANDER OR MINT LEAVES, SHREDDED
50G TOASTED FLAKED ALMONDS

PEEL the green bananas with a sharp knife (this isn't as easy as it is with ripe ones) and slice into 1cm discs.

HEAT the oil in a large saucepan, add the onion and fry over a medium heat for about 5 minutes until soft. Add the green bananas, curry paste and turmeric and fry for another minute or so until fragrant.

POUR in the coconut milk and bring to the boil, then stir in the red pepper, green beans, garlic and ginger, cover and simmer for 5 minutes. Season to taste with salt and pepper.

DIVIDE the curry among 4 serving bowls and serve sprinkled with the chillies, coriander or mint and almonds.

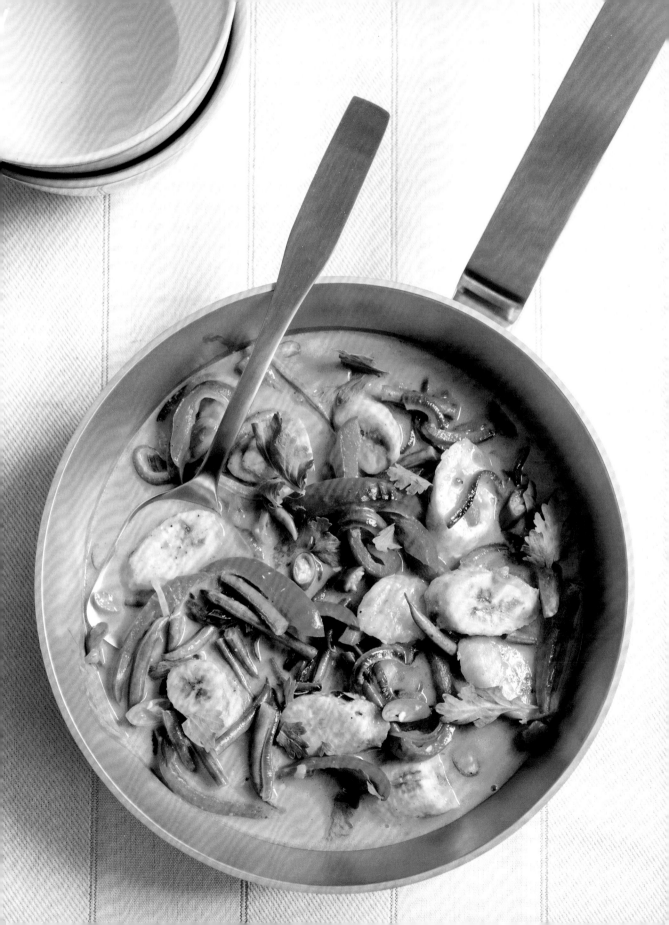

APPLES

Tasty, super-affordable and packed with benefits, apples have come a long way from their homelands in the wild forests of Kazakhstan to become one of the most popular fruit on the planet. It seems wherever they are eaten, they are also a common ingredient in traditional medicines, too. As I'm a total sucker for an old-school adage, I trawled the scientific literature to see if an apple a day really could keep the doctor away, and this is what I found.

♡ HEART DISEASE

In one small trial at the Ohio State University, consuming an apple a day resulted in an impressive 40 per cent drop in participants' LDL cholesterol within just 4 weeks, a difference similar to that between people with normal coronary arteries and sufferers of coronary heart disease. Now, although this trial used a tiny sample size of just 16 patients, its results were partially echoed by research at the University of Florida a year earlier, which found women consuming 75g of dried apple slices a day saw their LDL levels fall by 23 per cent after 3 months. Despite this sweet treat adding an extra 240 calories (roughly equivalent to a chocolate bar) to their daily diet, these women did not gain weight either, in fact they lost an average of 1.4kg.

Studies like these add to a wider body of clinical trials that have also reported apple consumption may indeed help modestly reduce LDL cholesterol levels, but usually to a much lesser extent and at doses closer to three apples a day. As research suggests that for every 1 per cent decrease in LDL cholesterol, there is a statistical 1 per cent decrease in incidences of cardiovascular events like heart attacks or strokes, falls like these could have a beneficial impact on your overall health.

♡ CANCER & DIABETES PREVENTION?

There is also evidence from population studies that links apple consumption with a reduced risk of developing certain cancers. Statistically, eating an apple (or more) a day appears to reduce incidence of throat cancer 41 per cent, colorectal cancer 30 per cent and both breast and ovarian cancer 24 per cent according to a review by Italian researchers. And it's not just cancer we see this pattern with either. A 2012 study from the Harvard School of Public Health found that consuming an apple a day was linked to a 35 per cent decrease in the risk of developing type 2 diabetes – which is on a par with the reduction seen with eating trendy 'superfood' blueberries. One long-running Australian study even found that consuming an apple a day was associated with a 35 per cent reduced risk of *all causes* of death in elderly women. Although population studies like these cannot prove a direct cause and effect relationship, merely point out statistical correlations, with stats like these, tossing an apple into your lunch box or gym bag could add up to quite a benefit.

♡ APPETITE CONTROL

Apples are an excellent source of fibre, and in particular a smooth, gel-like one called pectin. This has been demonstrated by a range of studies to help to slow digestion, creating the feeling of fullness. Scientists at the University of Pennsylvania, for example, reported that consuming the equivalent of two sliced apples 15 minutes before a meal could cut total calorie intake by 15 per cent (even after the calories in the apple were included). Faced with an all-you-can-eat spread, participants consumed an average of 180 calories fewer – about the number in a packet of crisps. Multiply that on a daily basis and in a few months this could really start to stack up!

Want to go one better? In this study, the apple slices were served peeled, a process that slashes their fibre content in half. Simply skipping this step will boost the fruit's potential to curb appetite.

🧺 THE HEALTHIEST APPLES GOING

An apple is an apple, is an apple. Simple, right? Actually, trials show there is a significant variation in the phytonutrient content of different apples, with some containing up to five times the antioxidant anthocyanins of others. Fortunately, the nutrition geeks at the University of Leeds have created a handy league table to help pick the best the greengrocer has to offer.

HIGHEST POLYPHENOLS

LOWEST POLYPHENOLS

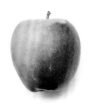

Polyphenols
475mg/100g

Braeburn

More antioxidants than any other variety in the trial, including a whopping one and a half times more polyphenols than Fuji, according to the University of Leeds. An excellent sweet/spicy crunch, according to me.

....

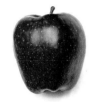

Polyphenols
444mg/100g

Red Delicious

Not my favourite for flavour – kind of dry and mealy – but it consistently ranks right at the top in studies for its outstanding polyphenol content. It seems, as with many fruit, in apples this is closely tied to colour. The redder, the better.

....

Polyphenols
410mg/100g

Pink Lady

Supersweet and aromatic, this modern variety now dominates many supermarkets. However, not all trials rank it so highly in the phyonutrient stakes as the Leeds team did.

....

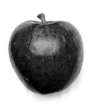

Polyphenols
375mg/100g

Royal Gala

There can be a large variation in phytonutrient content with Royal Gala, even between apples on the same tree. Pick the bright red ones for maximum benefit (see 'Two Apples from the Same Crate', page 114).

....

Polyphenols
373mg/100g

Granny Smith

This is tart, fresh and consistently reported as one of the highest antioxidant varieties going and the Leeds University study is no exception.

....

Polyphenols
368mg/100g

Bramley

The famed cooker isn't so bad in the nutritional stakes, but perhaps not once you simmer it up in an avalanche of sugar. Enjoy it for pleasure in pies and crumbles, but probably not for health.

....

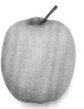

Polyphenols
343mg/100g

Golden Delicious

This apple comes out pretty low in almost all studies. In one trial its high sugar content and low phytonutrient levels were found not only not to reduce cholesterol, but also to slightly increase it. Maybe one to pass on given all the other great options?

....

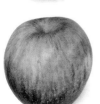

Polyphenols
330mg/100g

Fuji

According to the Leeds scientists, Fuji had a third less polyphenols than Braeburn. Usually ranked pretty low by the nutritional bean counters, although not all studies agree.

TWO APPLES FROM THE
SAME CRATE

Red apples are triggered into producing their characteristic colour by exposure to sunlight. As the UV rays hit their skins, the cells here react by churning out antioxidant pigments called anthocyanins to protect themselves from damage. As it's these same chemicals that are believed to confer many of their health benefits, simply picking the reddest in the crate will give you the most phytonutrients. If that weren't enough, research has shown redder apples can be over 10 per cent sweeter than paler ones of the same variety, even from the same tree!

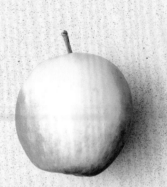

Significantly lower in anthocyanins. In fact as little as half.

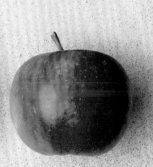

Colour shows anthocyanins are super-high here.

STORE 'EM ON THE SILL

Here's the weird thing, even once harvested it appears apples can still react to the ultraviolet rays in sunlight, generating loads more health benefits, at least according to the Norwegian University of Life Sciences. In fact, basking under UV lamps for 10 days could up to double the antioxidant levels in their skin and spike the vitamin C content here six times, without affecting their flavour. Plus, they look prettier on the windowsill than in the fridge, so why not?

FRESHER ISN'T ALWAYS BETTER

I am forever reading scare stories in the press about crops like apples – that instead of being fresh from the tree they can be *months* old before they get to you. Indeed, that is very true. So let's see what actually happens to their nutrient content in storage. A bunch of Polish food scientists, aiming to answer this question, mimicked the processes apples go through from farm to table. They stored two different varieties at 1°C for 4 months (as is done in commercial storage) and then took them out and kept them at room temperature for a week to simulate sitting on a supermarket shelf. They found that these apples actually experienced a 20 per cent *increase* in polyphenols and more than a doubling of their antioxidant content. This wasn't a freak one-off either, with very similar results reflected in at least two other trials.

DON'T BOTHER PEELING

Your mum was right, apple skins are indeed good for you. But you might be surprised to know by how much. Half of all the antioxidants, including vitamins A and C, plus an antioxidant called quercetin, are found in the skin, making 10 seconds of peeling all that is needed to slash levels of these key nutrients by as much as 50 per cent. Half of all the fibre in apples is found in the skin too so removing it can knock down fibre levels from 4.4g to just 2.1g per 100g – below the 3g amount needed to qualify as a 'good source of fibre'.

Peeling apples also significantly reduces the content of a group of compounds called triterpenoids that might show antitumour activity, according to a 2007 Cornell University study in human liver, colon and breast cancer cells (well, in test tubes, at least). This may be to do with the ability of apple peel extracts to 'turn on' a gene that suppresses tumours in our bodies, which is normally turned off in cancers in active growth. The researchers who made this finding concluded that 'apple peel extract possesses strong antiproliferative effects against cancer cells, and apple peels should not be discarded from the diet'. Do less work, get better nutrition and potentially even flick the switch on cancer cells? I call that a good deal.

NUKE THEM WITH ACID

So if peeling is bad news, you might assume the best type of apple is one as close to its raw, natural state as possible? Well, surprisingly, this just isn't the case, at least according to a team at the University of Warsaw. They found that lightly cooking apples with a quick blast of just a few minutes in the microwave or pan to make purée could double or even triple the levels of some of their of polyphenols. This was not only due to the cooking breaking down the cells in the skin, which allowed the nutrients trapped in the fibrous peel to escape, but also appeared to work by destroying an enzyme called polyphenol oxidase. This compound is the stuff that reacts with the oxygen in the air to make apples turn brown (oxidize) when you cut them, in so doing degrading their levels of these all-important polyphenols.

In addition to cooking, adding a little vitamin C powder to stop this browning made things even better, apparently. At home, a squirt of lemon juice over freshly cut apples will do the same thing, preserving more of their colour and health benefits. Incidentally, between pan cooking and microwave cooking, the superfast heating in the microwave was shown by the Warsaw team to degrade polyphenol oxidase a little faster, resulting in enhanced retention of the good stuff.

SCARLET 'SUPER APPLES'

Exciting breeding work is unleashing a new generation of red-fleshed apples, which can contain up to twice the polyphenols and five times the healthy anthocyanins of regular light-fleshed apples. Using traditional breeding methods, several teams around the world have been using wild apple varieties from their original home in the mountains of Kazakhstan to introduce genes that give them a gorgeous red hue and superior nutritional value.

The race is on, though, because many of these varieties are now under threat in their homeland because of forest clearance, showing how vital conservation work continues to be to the future of our food. Track them down in farmers' markets or, better yet, plant your very own tree. These varieties such as Redlove are sold by many garden catalogues for roughly the same price as boring old Bramley and can yield fruit in the very same year you plant them.

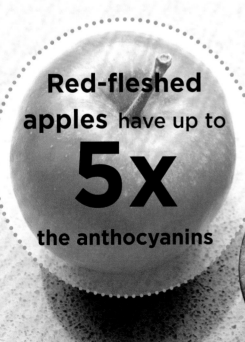

Red-fleshed apples have up to **5x** the anthocyanins

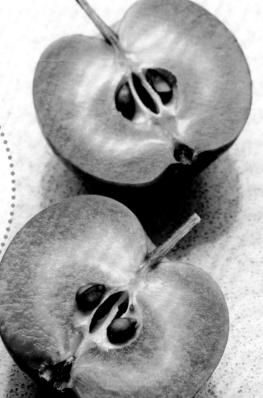

LEEK, POTATO & APPLE SOUP

OK, it's not the first combination that might spring to mind perhaps, but fresh apples make an excellent flavour pairing with classic leek and potato soup, adding a refreshing sweet-tart dimension and loads of phytonutrients. As warm and fuzzy as a woolly autumn jumper.

SERVES 4
PREP TIME 20 MINUTES
COOK TIME 45–60 MINUTES

....

1 TBSP BUTTER

1 TBSP OLIVE OIL

1 ONION, SLICED

3 LEEKS, TRIMMED, CLEANED AND SLICED

2 LARGE POTATOES, PEELED AND DICED

3 RED APPLES, QUARTERED, CORED AND SLICED

2.5CM PIECE OF FRESH ROOT GINGER, PEELED AND GRATED

2 GARLIC CLOVES, GRATED

1 TSP TURMERIC

750ML VEGETABLE OR CHICKEN STOCK

250ML WATER

100ML MILK

SALT AND PEPPER

NUT TOPPING

A LITTLE OLIVE OIL

50G WALNUTS, ROUGHLY CHOPPED

1 TBSP PUMPKIN SEEDS

SMALL PINCH OF CHILLI POWDER

1 RED APPLE, DICED

HEAT the butter and oil in a large saucepan, add the onion and leeks and cook gently for 5–10 minutes until softened. Add the potatoes, apples, ginger and garlic and cook for another 5 minutes until softened.

STIR through the turmeric and then add the stock, measured water and milk. Bring to the boil, then reduce the heat and simmer for 30–40 minutes, or until the vegetables are completely soft.

MEANWHILE, make the nut topping. Heat a little oil in a small nonstick frying pan, add the walnuts, pumpkin seeds and chilli powder and season with salt and pepper. Cook for about 5 minutes, stirring frequently, until the nuts are golden brown and toasted. Remove from the pan and leave to cool.

TAKE the soup off the heat, season with salt and pepper and blitz in the pan with a stick blender until smooth. Check the seasoning and reheat if necessary.

LADLE the soup into bowls and serve with the nut topping and diced apple sprinkled on top.

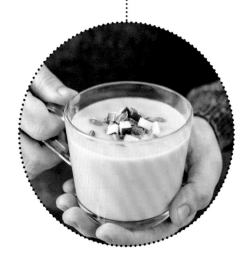

BAKED APPLE SKIN TWISTS

Still can't resist peeling apples for your next salad or smoothie? This recipe will transform former food scraps into crisp shards of surprisingly moreish appley goodness.

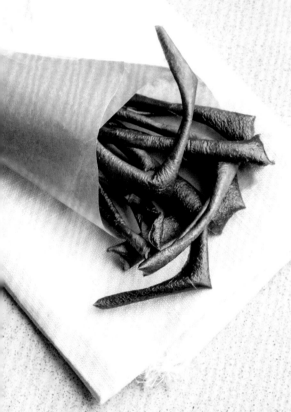

DON'T JUICE THEM

Juicing is a fad that seems to cycle in and out of health-food fashion. Aside from removing the vast majority of the fibre and upping the sugars gram for gram, studies have shown that juicing also removes many of the vitamins, minerals and other nutrients, which are left behind in the extracted pulp.

Run the juice through a filter or centrifuge, as many apple juice manufacturers do to get a crystal-clear result, and you reduce its polyphenol content by a whopping one and a half times that of traditional cloudy juice. In a 2013 Danish study, subjects drinking clear apple juice not only did not enjoy the 6.7 per cent reduction in their LDL cholesterol that was experienced by a group eating whole apples, but actually saw the exact opposite effect, with their levels of this 'bad' cholesterol increase by 6.9 per cent.

SERVES 2
PREP TIME 10 MINUTES
COOK TIME 1 HOUR

PEELED SKINS OF 4–5 RED APPLES

1 TSP LEMON JUICE

½ TSP GRANULATED SUGAR (OPTIONAL)

⅛ TSP GROUND CINNAMON

PREHEAT the oven to 120°C/Gas Mark ½.

PLACE the apple skins in a bowl, sprinkle over the lemon juice and sugar, if using, and toss to combine.

SCATTER the apple skins, skin-side down, over a large baking sheet and bake for about 1 hour until crisp. Dust lightly with cinnamon and you're away.

Apple juice can have as much as **88%** less antioxidant activity than whole apples

Cloudy apple juice contains up to **4x** the antioxidants of clear (but is still no match for eating the whole fruit)

STACKED APPLE CLUB SALAD

Probably my favourite quick lunch, this salad can be knocked together with leftover odds and sods. Sweet, crisp apples meet salty bacon and creamy blue cheese in an indulgent salad packed with healthy ingredients.

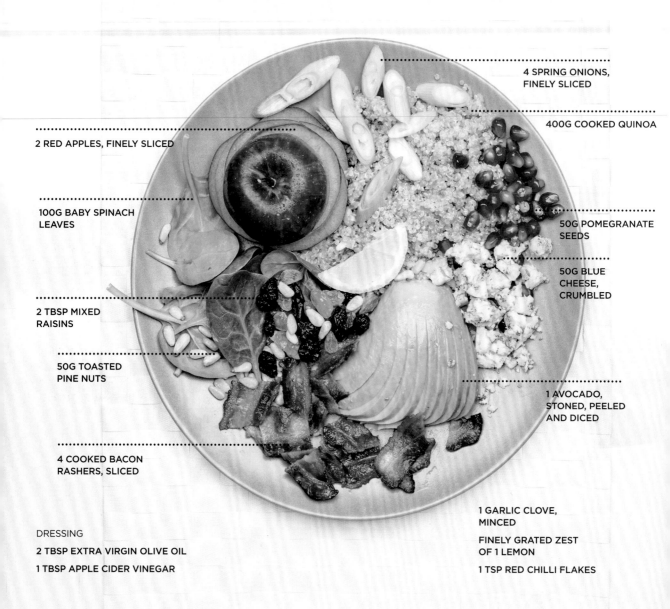

4 SPRING ONIONS, FINELY SLICED

400G COOKED QUINOA

2 RED APPLES, FINELY SLICED

100G BABY SPINACH LEAVES

50G POMEGRANATE SEEDS

50G BLUE CHEESE, CRUMBLED

2 TBSP MIXED RAISINS

50G TOASTED PINE NUTS

1 AVOCADO, STONED, PEELED AND DICED

4 COOKED BACON RASHERS, SLICED

1 GARLIC CLOVE, MINCED

FINELY GRATED ZEST OF 1 LEMON

1 TSP RED CHILLI FLAKES

DRESSING

2 TBSP EXTRA VIRGIN OLIVE OIL

1 TBSP APPLE CIDER VINEGAR

SERVES 4

PREP TIME ABOUT 30 MINUTES

PUT the cooked quinoa in a large salad bowl with 1 minced garlic clove, the finely grated zest of 1 lemon and 1 tsp red chili flakes and toss well. Add the remaining ingredients.

WHISK the dressing ingredients together in a small bowl, then drizzle over the salad.

APPLE CRUMBLE BIRCHER

The ultimate grab-and-go breakfast that'll give you the best nutritional start
(not to mention 15 minutes' extra lie-in time) every morning. Serve at home or on the go.
In the autumn I use red-fleshed apples from a potted tree on my patio, which gives the
whole mix a beautiful dusky pink colour and additional heart-healthy polyphenols. Yum.

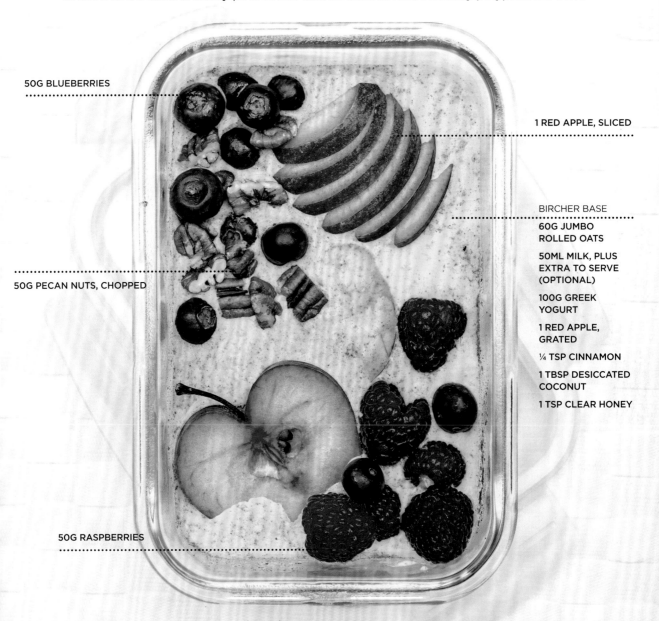

50G BLUEBERRIES

1 RED APPLE, SLICED

BIRCHER BASE

60G JUMBO ROLLED OATS

50ML MILK, PLUS EXTRA TO SERVE (OPTIONAL)

100G GREEK YOGURT

1 RED APPLE, GRATED

¼ TSP CINNAMON

1 TBSP DESICCATED COCONUT

1 TSP CLEAR HONEY

50G PECAN NUTS, CHOPPED

50G RASPBERRIES

SERVES 1
PREP TIME 10 MINUTES,
PLUS OVERNIGHT SOAKING

COMBINE all the bircher base ingredients in a plastic container, cover and leave to soak in the fridge overnight.

PREPARE the apple and pecans in the morning. Scatter the apples, blueberries, raspberries and pecans over the bircher base just before serving. You can always add a little extra milk, if you want a looser consistency.

INSTANT APPLE SUNDAE

This super-simple apple sundae can can be whizzed together in literally seconds from just five ingredients, too. No ice-cream maker needed!

Lighter and fresher tasting than regular ice cream, it's sky-high fruit content plus a healthy dose of protein and calcium from the creamy Greek yogurt means there is little room left for masses of fat and sugar. You can do the same thing with any fruit you fancy, too, from strawberries to mangoes and bananas.

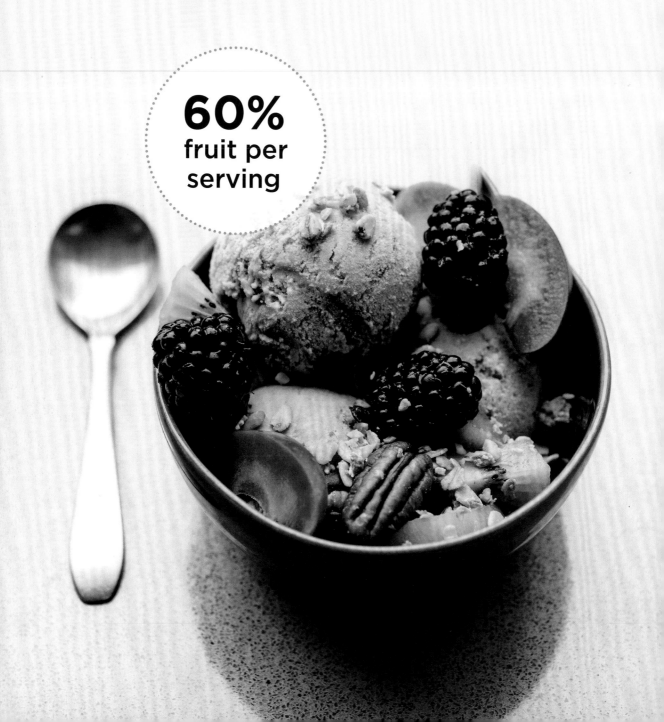

60% fruit per serving

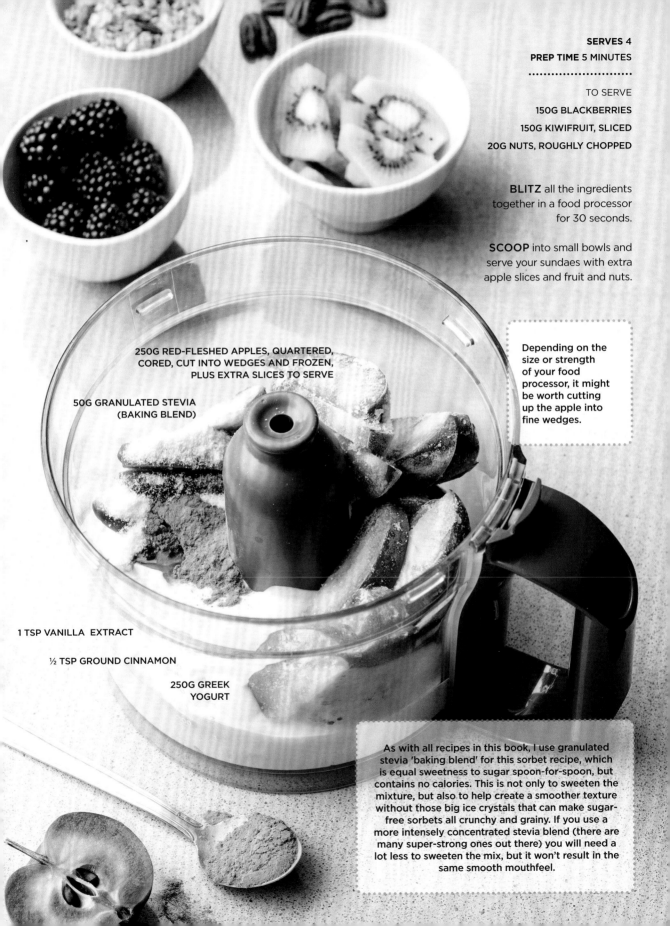

SERVES 4
PREP TIME 5 MINUTES

••••••••••••••••••••••••••

TO SERVE
150G BLACKBERRIES
150G KIWIFRUIT, SLICED
20G NUTS, ROUGHLY CHOPPED

BLITZ all the ingredients together in a food processor for 30 seconds.

SCOOP into small bowls and serve your sundaes with extra apple slices and fruit and nuts.

250G RED-FLESHED APPLES, QUARTERED, CORED, CUT INTO WEDGES AND FROZEN, PLUS EXTRA SLICES TO SERVE

50G GRANULATED STEVIA (BAKING BLEND)

Depending on the size or strength of your food processor, it might be worth cutting up the apple into fine wedges.

1 TSP VANILLA EXTRACT

½ TSP GROUND CINNAMON

250G GREEK YOGURT

As with all recipes in this book, I use granulated stevia 'baking blend' for this sorbet recipe, which is equal sweetness to sugar spoon-for-spoon, but contains no calories. This is not only to sweeten the mixture, but also to help create a smoother texture without those big ice crystals that can make sugar-free sorbets all crunchy and grainy. If you use a more intensely concentrated stevia blend (there are many super-strong ones out there) you will need a lot less to sweeten the mix, but it won't result in the same smooth mouthfeel.

BERRIES

Out of all fruit and veg, berries have undoubtedly attracted one of the largest collective bodies of scientific research, and with good reason. Aside from being a rich source of vitamins, minerals and fibre, their complex phytonutrient make-up (and in particular, the anthocyanin pigments that give them their red and purple coloration) is associated with a diverse array of health benefits. Here's what the latest research suggests consuming more of them could do for you.

♡ HEART HEALTH

Adding a large handful of blueberries (about 100g) to the daily diet of a group of middle-aged women appeared to quell blood pressure by 6 per cent according to researchers at Florida State University. This took them from a high 138/80 to well within the safe zone of 131/75. The women's arteries were also found to be measurably less stiff after just 2 months of enjoying a serving of blueberries a day. Even very modest amounts, say 3 small handfuls a week, could potentially make a big difference to your health, slashing the statistical risk of heart attack as much as 34 per cent according to one Harvard University study. Liberal berry consumption has also been associated with a reduction in harmful LDL cholesterol, raising healthy HDL cholesterol, as well as reducing chronic inflammation. And it can do it pretty quickly, too – in some studies, in as little as 4 weeks. Some impressive early stats. More research is underway to uncover more.

♡ BRAIN BOOST?

One of the quirky properties of anthocyanins is that, unlike the many other phytonutrients, they are able to cross the blood–brain barrier and accumulate in the areas that are essential for intelligence, at least in animal studies. When it comes to humans, the *Annals of Neurology* reports that in elderly participants, diets rich in berries were linked with a delay in cognitive ageing of 2.5 years, with the fruit appearing to slow the rate of mental decline.

But what if they could not only slow decline, but also potentially reverse it? Surely that would be too good to be true? Well, according to a very small trial by the USDA Human Nutrition Research Center on Aging, adding an average of 500ml (about 1½ glasses) of blueberry juice to the diets of older people with cognitive impairment could actually improve their performance in tests designed to assess certain forms of learning and memory, as well as easing symptoms of depression after just 3 months. Hardly ironclad proof for a berry-based wonder drug, but an intriguing result nonetheless, which has been echoed in other small-scale human studies.

♡ CANCER PREVENTION

As with many fruit and veg, there are loads of test-tube studies that suggest berries and their extracts might help fight the oxidative stress and inflammation in our bodies that can lead to certain types of cancer. They also appear capable of suppressing the growth of tumour cells in lab tests and animal models. But what about in the real world? What about in people? One trial by the Ohio State University aimed to answer just this question by investigating the effect of strawberry consumption in a phase 2 clinical trial with patients suffering from mild to moderate precancerous lesions of the throat. After consuming admittedly a huge amount of freeze-dried strawberries (equivalent to a large punnet or so of fresh fruit) each day for 6 months, 80 per cent of the patients saw their lesions either regress significantly or disappear altogether. This may sound astonishing, but the patients given a more realistic half that strawberry dose saw no significant benefit. Further trials are eagerly awaited.

♡ DIABETES & WEIGHT MANAGEMENT

Give a bunch of overweight female volunteers 100g of bilberries to eat every day for a month and what happens? Well, according to a small Finnish trial reported in the *European Journal of Clinical Nutrition*, a slight, but statistically significant decrease in waist circumference of 1.2cm (about half an inch) and even a slight reduction in weight, that's what. OK, so these stats aren't exactly mind-boggling, but considering the participants made no other changes in their lifestyle, this was a surprising finding. It also adds to a growing collection of studies from around the world that suggest that high berry intake may have a positive impact on diabetes and weight management, including by reducing blood sugars and calming inflammation.

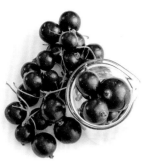

Anthocyanins
457mg/100g

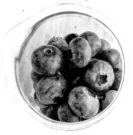

Anthocyanins
387mg/100g

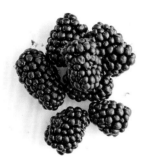

Anthocyanins
245mg/100g

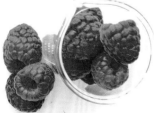

Anthocyanins
92mg/100g

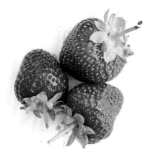

Anthocyanins
42mg/100g

HIGHEST ANTHOCYANINS

LOWEST ANTHOCYANINS

Blackcurrants

Sorry blueberries, you have been well and truly beaten in the phytonutrient stakes according to this ranking by the United States Department of Agriculture (USDA). With more than twice the anthocyanins (according to one trial at least) and a whopping 37 times the vitamin C, this old-school British berry really has the stats on its side. It's even up to 40 per cent richer in polyphenols and antioxidants, too. Although this can vary significantly between cultivars, blackcurrants consistently rank the highest of all berries for phytonutrient content across a range of studies. I just don't know why they aren't more popular.

Blueberries

The undisputed poster boy for the nutritional benefits of berries, and with great reason, too. Among the most commonly eaten fruit, they are second only to blackcurrants in their anthocyanin content, with over five times that of raspberries, for example. If you can track down wild ones they are even better (see 'Go Wild', page 124).

Blackberries

Blackberries might have fewer anthocyanins than blueberries according to most trials, but they are still an excellent source of these purple pigments. Some studies suggest they may also have higher total antioxidant activity, as much as four times more, in fact. So, poor relation they are not. Just like blueberries, the wild ones have consistently shown to be richer in phytonutrients than shop-bought. Plus, they are free! Get out and pick a load this autumn and bung them in the freezer to get a year-round supply of up to 35 per cent more of the good stuff in exchange for nothing more than enjoying some sunshine and fresh air, according to the University of Oslo.

Raspberries & strawberries

It's quite a leap down from blackberries to raspberries and strawberries in the anthocyanin stakes. You can tell that just by looking at their lighter colour. Raspberries have less than half the amount of blackberries, and strawberries half that again. Despite this, their total antioxidant activity still remains sky-high, broadly similar to that of blueberries and with loads more vitamin C. But why?

Well it turn out raspberries, along with blackberries, also happen to be one of the richest of all commonly eaten foods in an intriguing antioxidant called ellagic acid. Several promising test-tube and animal studies suggest this may help control the growth and spread of cancer cells. What about strawberries? They might contain about half that of raspberries and blackberries, but are still one of the richest dietary sources. So get tucking in.

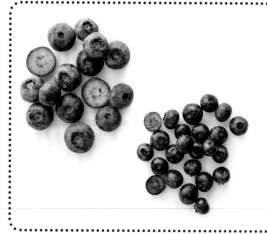

GO WILD

If you can get your hands on wild blueberries, these guys are even better, although exactly how much better does depend where in the world you live. Lowbush blueberries (marketed as 'wild blueberries' in North America) not only are more richly flavoured, but also contain one and a half times more anthocyanins, despite their small size. However, even these pale in comparison to the wild European bilberry, popular in eastern Europe and Scandinavia, which has a whopping four times more anthocyanins than the regular cultivated blueberry. Both types are usually sold frozen rather than fresh, but this should have little impact on their phytonutrient content (see 'Freeze-framing Nutrition', below).

CHEAPER CAN BE BETTER

It is no coincidence that smaller blueberries are richer in anthocyanins, as these purple pigments are found almost exclusively in the skin. The smaller the berry, the larger the surface area and, in turn, the more skin they contain gram for gram. That means the 'value' brand blueberries in supermarkets, which are just the runty ones that never get selected for the more 'premium' packs (despite often being from the exact same variety, country of origin and even farm!), can be measurably higher in phytonutrients, not to mention about 40 per cent cheaper.

FORGET THE FRIDGE

When it comes to berries, fresher isn't always better. You see, once many berries are picked from the plant they can continue to ripen, becoming darker in colour, more aromatic and richer in a range of phytonutrients. According to the *Journal of Agricultural and Food Chemistry*, this is certainly the case for strawberries, whose anthocyanins can quadruple a week after harvest, giving them 50 per cent more antioxidants to boot. All this goes hand in hand with a spike in aroma chemicals (the stuff that gives strawberries their characteristic flavour) and a deepening in colour, so it's a winner all round really. Raspberries and blueberries show similar results, too, after just a matter of days. The chemical reactions that trigger these changes occur best at room temperature (20°C) and are significantly hampered when chilled below 10°C. So simply plonking your punnet of berries on the work surface rather than storing it in the fridge could make for measurably tastier, healthier results within just a day or two. Remember, though, these berries will already have taken a few days to get to you, so keep an eye on them. Their phytonutrients tend to peak just before the mould sets in. Don't say I didn't warn you.

FREEZE-FRAMING NUTRITION

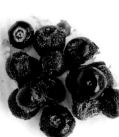

Miles cheaper, super-convenient and always in season, frozen berries have a lot going for them, but how do they stack up in terms of nutrition? Well, here's more good news: there has actually been a load of research on this and it turns out that putting them on ice has essentially zero effect on their nutritional value, at least for strawberries and raspberries, with blueberries only decreasing after many months of storage. In my local supermarket, frozen berries are less than half the price of fresh, so going for the easy option can also get you twice the bang for your buck.

GOOD NEWS, PUDDING LOVERS!

It turns out not only are the phytonutrients in berries surprisingly heat stable, cooking may even cause them to shoot up significantly. This means compotes, pies and jellies could be just as good if not better for you than the fresh fruit, in the antioxidant stakes at least. Hallelujah!

As always, it appears it is all about how long you cook them for that is key. In one study, published in the journal *Food Control,* an international team of researchers found that baking or boiling blueberries for under 30 minutes had a negligible impact on their antioxidant capacity, as did whacking them in the microwave for 3 minutes. Only when baking or boiling time was raised to 30–60 minutes or nuking to 5 minutes (quite a long time in a microwave) did they see a significant decrease. Other studies have found that although the total anthocyanin content does dip slightly, the total level of antioxidants and polyphenols remained stable during cooking.

In fact, a brief blast of heat by sautéeing them over a medium flame has been shown in several trials to trigger a spike in nutrition, as much as doubling their antioxidants and tripling their polyphenol content in one study by Oregon Health Sciences University. Now, where's my pudding bowl?

BERRIES & CARBS

There is a growing body of evidence that suggests one of the mechanisms behind how berry consumption may benefit health is through their effect on digestion – particularly that of high-carb, high-fat foods. In test-tube trials, extracts of berries have been shown to suppress the action of the enzymes our bodies use to break down and absorb carbs and fats – even in the relatively tiny quantities that would reach the gut.

But what about in our bodies? Well, in one trial published in the *British Journal of Nutrition* participants were given a high-carb, moderate-fat meal, designed to spike their blood sugar and trigger inflammation, along with either a strawberry-based drink or a placebo drink. Chronic inflammation that results from diets like this is linked to obesity, diabetes and even the development of cancer. The group that consumed the strawberry drink had not only a far lower insulin response, but also a 25 per cent reduction in one of the measures of inflammation. At least four other studies have echoed these potentially protective effects when berries were consumed with white bread, rye bread, sugary cornflakes and even with straight-up table sugar. Although strawberries and raspberries appear to be much more effective than other species – reducing the impact of the carbs by over a third – weirdly, a mix of various berries had a similar effect, suggesting there may have been a synergistic reaction taking place. Theoretically, this *could* mean they may help keep you fuller for longer, reduce the risk of diabetes and even cause you to store less of what you eat as fat. *Theoretically*.

Before you get carried away, it would be remiss of me not to point out that at least one trial found that adding berries to pancakes had no impact whatsoever on the after-effects of carby indulgence. Clearly, there is so much more to discover around what it is about berries that may cause this effect – if there is an effect – but in the meantime I for one will be chucking them on everything.

BERRIES & DAIRY

Now for some rather inconvenient news. A range of studies is beginning to point to the idea that milk, and specifically milk protein, may bind to anthocyanins and therefore prevent their absorption by the body.

In one, admittedly very small, clinical trial at Italy's National Institute for Food and Nutrition Research, blending blueberries with milk instead of water completely blocked their ability to raise the levels of antioxidants in the blood of participants, even several hours after consumption. These findings were echoed by another study in the *International Journal of Food Sciences and Nutrition*, which suggested that adding milk to oats and blueberries decreased some anthocyanin pigments to undetectable levels. In one experiment, combining strawberries with yogurt led to an immediate decrease in their total antioxidant activity by 23 per cent, with levels of some anthocyanins slashed in half after 24 hours. But it isn't just anthocyanins – adding milk to blackberries has also been shown to block the absorption of the potentially cancer-quelling ellagic acid they are so rich in.

So, what about the alternatives? Well, at least one trial has tested the effect soya milk may have. And guess what? Fruit smoothies made with soya milk exhibited significantly more antioxidant capacity than those made with water. This could mean that swapping yogurt and milk for soya or nut-based alternatives not only might add more healthy plant-based protein to your diet, but could even improve the good stuff in the berries. I feel, for me personally at least, it's a simple swap that's often worth the potential benefit. Although goodness knows, even I don't stick rigidly to my own rules!

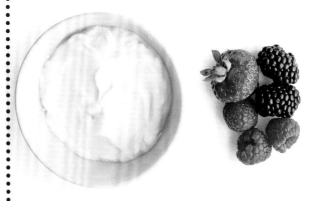

SUMMER PUDDING

Traditional English summer pudding is to me an instant flashback to the smell of cut lawn, the sun on your face and lazy days in the garden. The best bit is it just happens to be 75 per cent fruit with only a tiny amount of sugar compared to other desserts. You can even dispense with this altogether and use stevia instead. Making this with frozen berries gives you the same nutrition at far lower cost, too. Boom!

SERVES 8

PREP TIME 30 MINUTES, PLUS OVERNIGHT CHILLING

....

7–8 VERY THICK SLICES OF WHITE BREAD, CRUSTS REMOVED

900G FROZEN SUMMER BERRIES

4 TBSP CASTER SUGAR OR GRANULATED STEVIA (BAKING BLEND)

FINELY GRATED ZEST OF 1 LEMON

TO SERVE

FRESH BERRIES

FLAKED ALMONDS

LINE a large pudding basin with 2 sheets of cling film. Cut a slice of the bread to fit the top of the basin, then cut a second slice of bread to fit the bottom of the basin. Line the bottom of the basin with the small circle of bread, then line the sides of the basin with the 6 remaining slices of bread, overlapping them a little.

TIP the frozen berries into a large saucepan, along with the sugar or stevia and lemon zest. Cook over low heat for 5–10 minutes until the mixture begins to lightly bubble.

SPOON the warm fruit mixture into the lined basin, reserving a cupful of the fruit mixture. (Leave the reserved fruit mixture to cool completely and then chill overnight.)

PLACE the large circle of bread on top of the filled pudding, cover with clingfilm, then top the pudding with a snug-fitting plate and weigh it down with a heavy can or packet. Leave the pudding to cool completely and then chill overnight.

TIP the pudding out on to a plate and pour over the reserved fruit mixture. Serve scattered with fresh berries and flaked almonds.

GOING NUTS WITH BERRIES

A recent review of the evidence behind the potential health benefits of berries in the *American Journal of Clinical Nutrition* reported: 'There is growing evidence that the synergy and interaction of all of the nutrients and other bioactive components in nuts and berries can have a beneficial effect on the brain and cognition.'

In particular, a compound found in nuts called phytic acid has been shown in some Japanese studies to help prevent the degradation of anthocyanins in berries, which can dramatically improve their bioavailability by as much as 1,500 per cent, in lab rats at least. As nuts, especially walnuts and almonds, are by far the richest everyday dietary sources of phytic acid, the amounts in an average serving also realistically reflect the concentrations used in the study. What's more, nuts and berries taste great together, so combining them is not exactly culinary hardship.

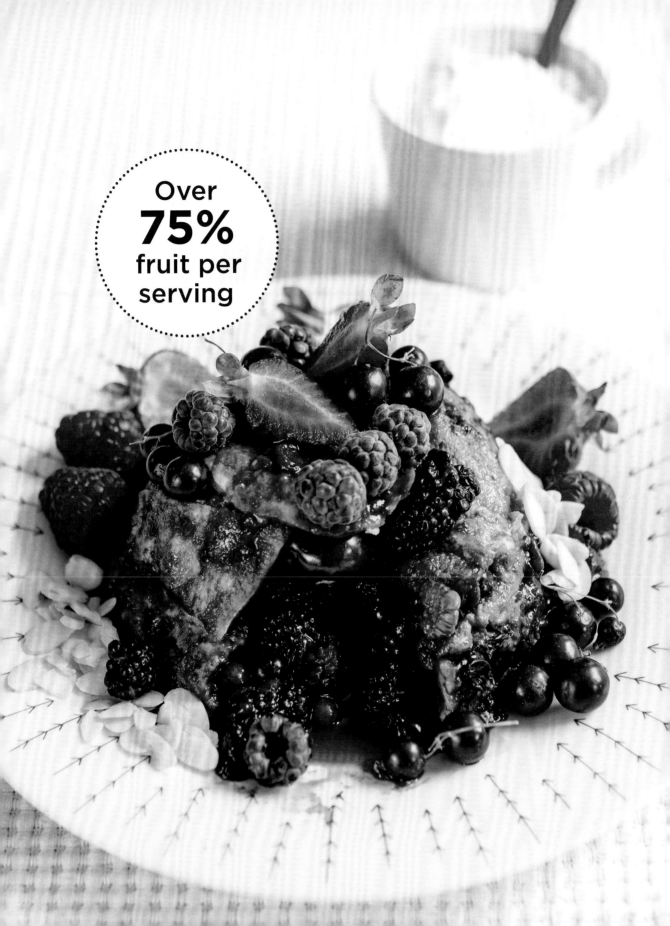

Over **75%** fruit per serving

5-MINUTE BLUEBERRY COMPOTE

This super-quick compote can be knocked up from scratch in about 5 minutes and, in the process, boosts the availability of health-promoting compounds in the blueberries. You can even save yourself a bit of money by using frozen blueberries – just add 2 minutes to the cooking time. Arrowroot creates a perfectly clear compote, but if you can't find it, plain old cornflour will thicken it just as well.

MAKES 300G

PREP TIME 2 MINUTES

COOK TIME 3 MINUTES

....

300G FRESH BLUEBERRIES

1 TBSP ARROWROOT OR CORNFLOUR

1 TSP MIXED SPICE

1 TSP GRANULATED STEVIA (BAKING BLEND)

FINELY GRATED ZEST AND JUICE OF 1 LEMON

PUT all the ingredients into a microwaveable bowl and mix well.

MICROWAVE on high for 3 minutes, stirring halfway through the cooking time. Leave to cool slightly before serving.

STORE the compote in the fridge for up to 1 week.

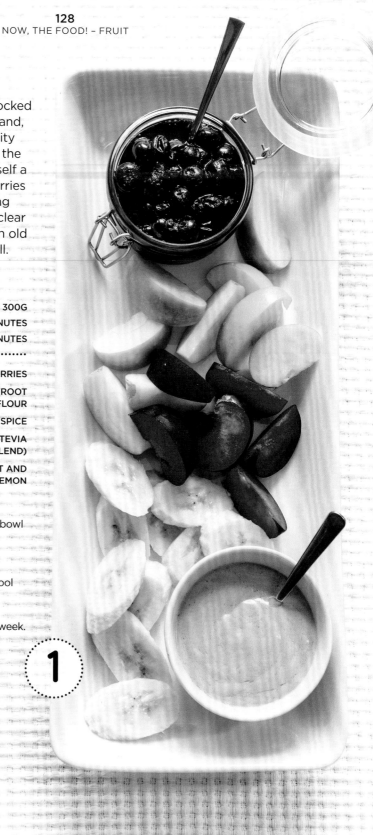

1

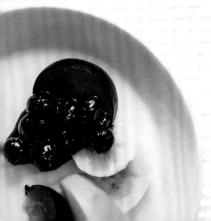

HOW TO SERVE

1 FRUIT WITH PEANUT BUTTER & JELLY DIPS

Spoon the **Blueberry Compote** into a ramekin or serving bowl. To make the peanut butter dip, mix together 2 tbsp **peanut butter** and 2 tbsp **water**, then transfer to another ramekin. Serve the dips with **fresh fruit** arranged on a serving platter.

2 BAKED FRENCH TOAST

Whisk together 2 **eggs**, 200ml **milk**, the finely grated zest and juice of 1 **orange**, 1 tsp **cinnamon**, 2 tbsp **clear honey** and 1 tsp **vanilla extract** in a large, shallow dish. Soak 4 thick slices of **wholegrain bread** in the mixture for 1–2 minutes, or until most of the liquid has been absorbed. Carefully transfer the bread to a greased large baking sheet and bake in a preheated oven, 200°C/Gas Mark 6, for about 25 minutes until golden. Serve with the **Blueberry Compote** and **fresh berries**.

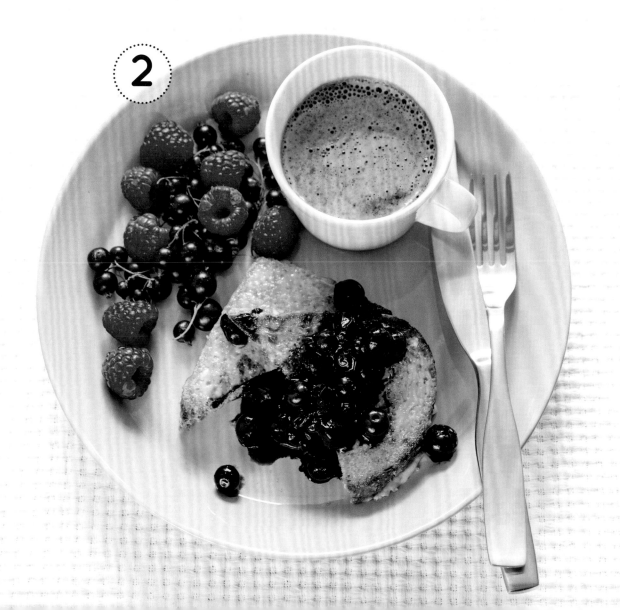

'ACAI-LESS' BOWL

My home-grown take on trendy acai bowls, which swaps the fruit
of this tropical palm with juicy, ripe blackcurrants.

SERVES 1

PREP TIME 5 MINUTES

....

100G STRAWBERRIES, HULLED, PLUS EXTRA TO
SERVE (OPTIONAL)

100G BLACKCURRANTS

2 SLICED BANANAS, FROZEN

150ML APPLE JUICE

1 THUMB-SIZED PIECE OF FRESH ROOT GINGER,
PEELED AND GRATED

TOPPINGS

A MIX OF FRUIT AND NUTS, PLUS MAYBE
A SNEAKY SQUARE OR THREE OF CHOCOLATE
AS A TREAT

BLITZ all the ingredients together in a
food processor or blender until you have
a smooth purée.

POUR the mixture into a serving bowl
and serve with your chosen toppings.

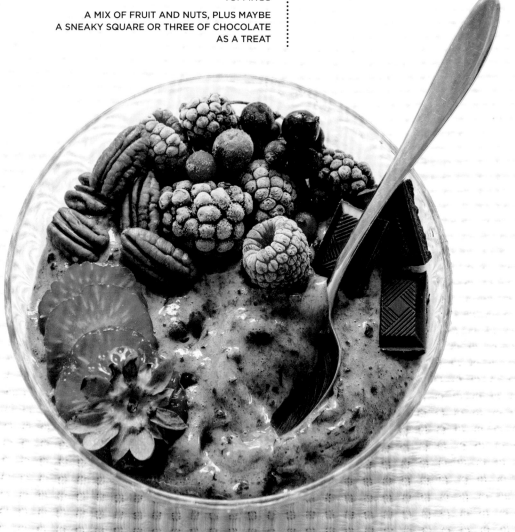

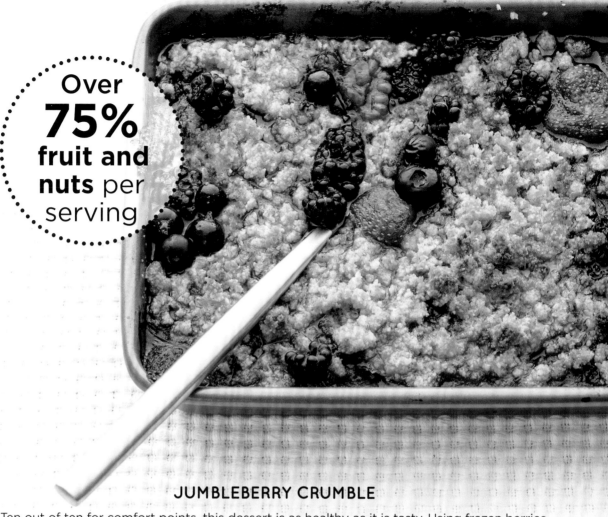

Over 75% fruit and nuts per serving

JUMBLEBERRY CRUMBLE

Ten out of ten for comfort points, this dessert is as healthy as it is tasty. Using frozen berries will give you the same nutrition for roughly half the price. Why not?

SERVES 4
PREP TIME 15 MINUTES
COOK TIME 30-35 MINUTES

500G MIXED FRESH BERRIES
¼ TSP CINNAMON
1 TBSP GRANULATED STEVIA (BAKING BLEND),
OR TO TASTE
2 TBSP CORNFLOUR
FINELY GRATED ZEST AND JUICE OF 1 LEMON

TOPPING
60G JUMBO OATS
60G GROUND ALMONDS
60G GRANULATED STEVIA (BAKING BLEND)
60G COLD UNSALTED BUTTER, DICED

PREHEAT the oven to 190°C/Gas Mark 5.

BLITZ all the topping ingredients together in a food processor – the final consistency should be a coarse rubble rather than a fine powder.

MIX the berries, cinnamon, stevia, cornflour, lemon zest and juice together in a separate bowl, then tip into a baking dish. Sprinkle the topping over the fruit.

BAKE for 30–35 minutes, or until the crumble is golden and crisp. Serve hot.

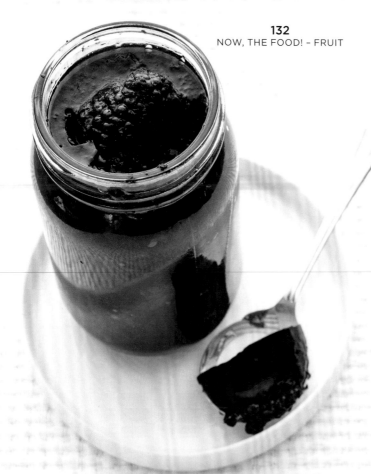

Growing your own blackberries? Well here's a nice coincidence: thornless varieties tend to have far more anthocyanins than varieties with thorns – in fact, on average twice as much, according to the *Journal of Agricultural and Food Chemistry*.

BLACKBERRY & CABERNET FREEZER JAM

Freezer jams are preserved by icy temperatures rather than sky-high sugar content and don't require prolonged boiling to ensure a good set. This means far less degradation of phytonutrients and far fewer calories, along with the convenient fact that they are also far easier to make. To me, it's win-win all round.

MAKES 500G

PREP TIME 10 MINUTES, PLUS OVERNIGHT CHILLING

COOK TIME 5 MINUTES

500G BLACKBERRIES

5 TBSP GRANULATED STEVIA (BAKING BLEND), PLUS EXTRA TO TASTE

A PINCH OF SALT

250ML CABERNET SAUVIGNON

3 TBSP AGAR FLAKES (USUALLY FOUND IN HEALTH-FOOD STORES AND THE BAKING SECTIONS OF SOME SUPERMARKETS)

TIP the blackberries, stevia and salt into a heatproof bowl and crush together with the back of a fork to create a chunky pulp.

POUR the wine into a small saucepan and scatter over the agar flakes. Slowly bring to a simmer, swirling the pan (not stirring) to help the flakes dissolve, then simmer gently for a minute or two until all the flakes have dissolved.

ADD the crushed berries to hot wine mixture, stir well to combine and simmer for 2–3 minutes. Taste for sweetness and add more stevia, if you like, then spoon into small freezer-proof plastic containers and leave to cool.

CHILL in the fridge overnight to allow the mixture to set. The jam will keep in the fridge for up to 1 week or small batches of the jam can be frozen for up to 1 year.

BREAKFAST YOGURT POPS

A handy, wholesome breakfast on the go, these are perfect for kids as they dash out the door.

MAKES 6 POPS

PREP TIME 10 MINUTES, PLUS FREEZING

....

300G MIXED BERRIES

2 TBSP GRANULATED STEVIA (BAKING BLEND)

300G GREEK YOGURT

2 TBSP HONEY, PLUS EXTRA FOR DRIZZLING

GRANOLA, FOR COATING

PLACE the berries and stevia in a microwavable bowl and microwave on high for 3 minutes, Stir to combine.

SPOON the berry mixture into 6 ice lolly moulds, followed by the yogurt and freeze for 6 hours.

REMOVE the ice lollies from the moulds, drizzle honey over each one, then dip into granola to coat.

You may have noticed I have combined dairy and berries here, despite flagging up emerging evidence suggesting the fruit's benefits might be quelled by milk protein on page 125. What can I say? I don't believe in slavish devotion to rules, even my own. After all, food is about enjoyment! These are so tasty they are worth a breaking a rule or two.

VARIATIONS

1 TROPICAL

Make the pops as left, replacing the berries with 250g puréed **mango** and the pulp of 2 **passion fruit**, and the granola with **desiccated coconut**.

2 APRICOT & PISTACHIO

Make the pops as left, replacing the berries with 300g chopped ripe **apricots**, and the granola with chopped **pistachios**.

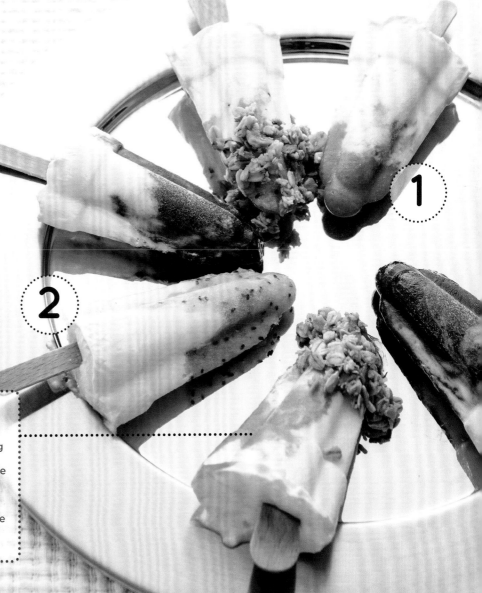

CITRUS

In a world of acai elixirs and goji granola, the humble orange might not ever grab headlines as 'superfood' *du jour*. But if it's health benefits backed by solid science you are after, citrus has it in droves. Easily one of the most nutrient-dense options on the produce aisle, trust me, there is far more to the world of citrus than a bit of vitamin C.

♡ REDUCED CANCER RISK?

Study after study has reported a strong link between regular citrus consumption and a reduced incidence of certain types of cancer, cutting the statistical risk of developing breast cancer 10 per cent, bladder cancer about 20 per cent and throat cancer a whopping 47 per cent among avid citrus scoffers. Now, of course, this is perhaps simply because citrus eaters might tend to consume more fruit and veg in general, exercise more or otherwise live healthier lifestyles, but the correlation is strikingly consistent nonetheless.

The underlying cause behind this *apparent* protective ability is still unknown. Keen to learn more, a team of Italian scientists set out to investigate the effects of a group of antioxidants called flavones, commonly found in citrus fruit, on the growth of lung cancer cells in lab rats. The authors reported a 'remarkable reduction' in the proliferation of cancers, with the flavones suppressing tumour growth by as much as 70 per cent, leading to a doubling in the life expectancy of the rats with terminal cancer. While this research is still in its infancy and many more trials are needed before we know whether these findings are transferable in human patients, when steely-faced lab geeks use words like 'remarkable' in scientific journals, it means the results frankly blew their minds.

One potential explanation for the apparent cancer-fighting capacity of citrus flavones is their ability to be easily absorbed by the body and persist in the blood for an unusual length of time – up to 24 hours according to some trials. Eat them every day and you have a continuous supply floating around in your system, helping to calm inflammation and mop up free radicals. Compared to other natural anticarcinogens such as the polyphenols in green tea or chocolate, which remain active in the body for just 4–6 hours, this gives flavones far more time to get to work.

♡ HEART PROTECTION

There are two different flavones that are uniquely found in citrus fruit: naringin (mainly found in grapefruit) and hesperidin (mainly in oranges). Eating either of these natural antioxidants has been shown by research to help significantly improve circulation – in fact, in as little as an hour after consumption. In one study at Japan's National Institute of Health Sciences, researchers put a group of women who

LOWEST ANTIOXIDANTS

Lemons & limes

Oranges

Grapefruit

were especially sensitive to cold in a freezing cold, refrigerated room to test the effects of plummeting temperature on the circulation. After sitting for ages in these icy conditions, unsurprisingly the women in the placebo group saw the temperature of their fingertips drop by just over 5°C. Yet those given a drink containing hesperidin just an hour before experienced less than half that fall, demonstrating significantly improved circulation to their extremities. The fingers of these poor women even regained normal temperature much more quickly after their hands were plunged into ice water by researchers. Scientists can be such kind souls!

OK, so a glass of OJ or two *might* just help keep your hands warm on a long winter walk, but what if the effects could extend much further? After all, studies suggest men and women with diets rich in citrus fruit also have almost half the risk of developing cardiovascular disease. Clinical trials have shown that consuming grapefruit and its extracts can also result in a significant decrease in systolic blood pressure of 2.43 mmHg and reduce 'bad' LDL cholesterol by 20 per cent in as little as 4 weeks. Take up the citrus habit and your heart might just thank you for it.

BRAIN FOOD

Citrus flavones have also attracted the attention of researchers for their anti-inflammatory properties and unusual ability to cross the blood–brain barrier, a highly selective structure that blocks over 98 per cent of drugs from reaching the brain. With many degenerative neurological diseases like Alzheimer's and Parkinson's being characterized by inflammation, this is an exciting combination of properties. For this reason, a growing collection of studies has sought to investigate the potential value

HIGHEST ANTIOXIDANTS

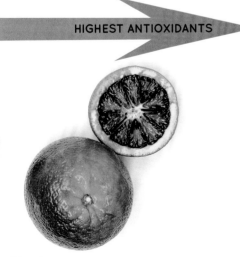

Blood oranges

of citrus flavones on brain health and has already yielded some pretty intriguing results.

In one German trial, lab mice exhibiting symptoms similar to Alzheimer's showed significant improvements in their social interaction and ability to carry out day-to-day behaviours such as nesting after just 10 days of being fed citrus extracts. Blood tests on these animals showed a significant reduction in the inflammation of the brain and slowing of the growth of the plaques that are typically found in the brains of patients with Alzheimer's.

In other animal trials, researchers noted that citrus extracts could prevent the death of brain cells brought about by neurotoxin poisoning that mimicked the effect of Alzheimer's in rats, with others showing it could even *reverse* learning and memory deficits that resulted. With test-tube studies also reporting a potential protective effect of citrus extracts against neurotoxins on cultured cells, several authors have concluded that these fruit could show promise in the future development of drugs and therapeutic foods to combat degenerative brain diseases. It's still a very long way from a cure, but a fascinating start!

MEMORY BOOST?

Even in healthy individuals, a number of small, short-term trials have provided early indications that eating citrus fruit may help improve memory and mental function. In one trial at the University of Reading, a group of healthy older participants who drank 500ml of orange juice each day for 8 weeks showed a small but significant 8 per cent improvement in memory tests. Put into context, in one of the tests subjects were required to learn a 'shopping list' of 15 words and recall them after about half an hour. In this test, an 8 per cent improvement would equate to remembering one more item in the list. According to the authors of the study, such small improvements in the short 8 weeks trial period 'could translate into substantial improvements over the lifespan'. It was hypothesized that this effect could be caused by the flavones in the juice improving blood flow to the brain and facilitating the transmission of information between brain cells. In another trial, the same research team went even further, reporting that a single 240ml dose of orange juice could significantly boost mental alertness and accuracy in psychological tests in healthy, middle-aged men, with the effects persisting for 6 hours after consumption. OK, so both these studies used a comparatively tiny sample size (the latter included only 24 men) and crucially were funded by a leading orange juice manufacturer; however, I can't wait to see what further research will uncover. In the meantime, swigging the OJ before your next exam couldn't hurt.

STORE BLOOD ORANGES IN THE COLD

Ever notice how in a batch of blood oranges some are far darker than others? This is because they start life looking just like regular oranges and are only triggered to produce their protective red anthocyanin pigments when exposed to winter chills, which is also why they tend to get redder as the season progresses. Luckily, this is really easy to mimic at home by just popping them in the fridge. Italian researchers found that the levels of anthocyanins in blood oranges stored at 4°C (typical domestic fridge temperature) skyrocketed to 8 times their original levels after just 6 days. Better still, the flavones and overall antioxidant activity were also raised and these levels remained high for several weeks afterwards, so you don't have to rush to eat them. Eight times the good stuff for zero work? Not a bad deal really. Interestingly, the same research also showed that regular oranges had an overall increase in antioxidants and vitamin C, but with a decrease in flavones, so the evidence of such a positive benefit for all oranges is less clear.

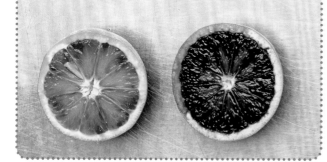

Red grapefruit have

34x

the **vitamin A** of **white ones**, and they **taste sweeter** too

LEMONS & LIMES

These are the citrus with the lowest levels of the antioxidant carotenes that give oranges and some grapefruits their rich colour and associated health benefits. And, while gram for gram they have a similar amount of vitamin C and flavones to sweet oranges, the intense acidity of lemons and limes also means we tend to consume them in much smaller amounts (a typical 1 tablespoon serving of lemon juice is 14 times smaller than a standard 250ml serving of orange juice). Tasty, yes, but not the most nutritious members of the family.

NAVEL ORANGES, MANDARINS, TANGERINES & SATSUMAS

All orange-coloured citrus are packed with good stuff. However, the deep pink flesh of the recently introduced Cara Cara variety has a slight edge, coming with 30 per cent more vitamin A than a regular navel orange and 20 per cent more vitamin C. Its stunning colour is the result of the presence of the antioxidant lycopene (see page 22) and enhanced amounts of betacarotene, which research suggests may protect against certain cancers. And to top it all off, it is less acid than many conventional oranges, which makes it perfect for those with sensitive tummies. Seek out these beauties in their winter season.

While regular oranges are higher in vitamin C and heart-healthy flavones, when it comes to the carotenes, mandarin varieties have the extra edge. Spanish research found that mandarins and clementines were markedly higher in these antioxidant pigments than sweet oranges and grapefruit, giving a deeper orange hue and three times the vitamin A of other citrus. Picking citrus with the deepest colour can reap nutritional dividends.

GRAPEFRUIT

Grapefruit are rich in naringin, a different type of flavone to the hesperidin found in oranges. While this may give them their unique health benefits, it also makes them taste bitter, which can put many people off enjoying them. It is, incidentally, this same chemical that causes the notorious 'Grapefruit Juice Effect', which can interfere with how certain medications, such as statins, are absorbed.

Not a fan of bitterness? Well, I have good news. Pink and red varieties of grapefruit are noticeably sweeter than the traditional white forms while at the same time (perhaps counterintuitively) containing similar levels of flavones. In fact, some modern bright red varieties like Star Ruby have been shown to have significantly more of these, containing up to twice the naringin of old-school white cultivars like Duncan. Not only that, but red and pink grapefruit come enriched with a whopping 34 times the vitamin A of the white varieties. In practical terms, this means eating just one medium red grapefruit could provide you with 50 per cent of your daily dose of vitamin A, compared with less than 2 per cent in the white kind.

But what about their effect on heart health? One study in the *Journal of Agricultural and Food Chemistry* decided to find out, putting red and white grapefruit to a head-to-head test. Researchers gave a group of patients with coronary artery disease either one red or white grapefruit to eat each day. After 30 days, all the grapefruit eaters saw significant falls in both their total cholesterol and in particular their levels of 'bad' LDL cholesterol. However, those eating the red variety fared twice as well, with their LDL cholesterol dropping by 20 per cent (compared to just 10.7 per cent eating the white variety). The red grapefruit group also experienced a drop in their levels of blood triglycerides – a key risk factor in developing heart disease. Those eating the white grapefruit showed no such benefit. The researchers concluded that this was due to the red variety's 'higher levels of bioactive compounds and significantly higher antioxidant potential'. Better flavour, prettier colour and enhanced nutrition? I know which one is going in my basket.

BLOOD ORANGES

These are unusual varieties of orange whose unique genetics trigger them to produce blood-red anthocyanin pigments (the same group of chemicals thought to give red wine and blueberries their health benefits) when exposed to low temperatures. Nutritionally, these guys are real superstars, containing up to 80 per cent more polyphenols, two and a half times the flavones and five times the antioxidant activity of a regular navel orange with a comparable amount of vitamin C. Research has demonstrated that a daily (albeit very large) 500ml glass of blood orange juice for as little as 7 days could help reduce inflammation, and in 8 weeks lower LDL cholesterol and blood pressure and raise antioxidant levels in the blood. For the greatest benefits seek out the darkest red Moro variety, which is far higher in phytonutrients than the red-specked Tarocco and Sanguinello varieties.

CHEAPER OJ IS BETTER

Over 50 per cent of all the world's oranges go to make juice, but a subtle twist on how it is made can have a dramatic effect on its potential health benefits. By going for comminuted orange juice over traditionally squeezed, studies suggest you could get juice with three times the antioxidant activity and over seven times the flavonoids – some pretty jaw-dropping stats! That is because comminuted juice, a technique used by many of the cheapest brands, blitzes up whole oranges to a pulp and then filters off the pulp, instead of slicing and squeezing oranges. During this process, chemicals from the nutrient-rich zest and skin leach into the juice, enhancing its nutritional composition. Who says the fanciest brands are always the healthiest?

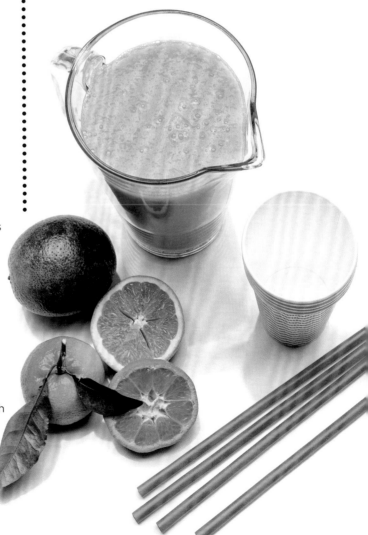

WHICH BIT IS BEST?

As with many fruit and veg, the nutrients in citrus are not distributed evenly across their tissues, but are tend to be more concentrated at their surface. In fact, the zest and pith found in citrus skins have consistently been shown to contain significantly higher levels of key antioxidants than the juice contained within, which means that we are often ironically throwing away the most nutritious bit of the fruit. Learning how to eat the *whole* orange gives you far more benefits. Let me explain.

Zest

The brightly coloured, aromatic zest of citrus might only make up a tiny part of the fruit, but it accounts for over a third of the vitamin C, being a richer source of carotenes than any other part.

Pith

The spongy white pith that makes up most of the skin contains a whopping 17 times the antioxidant activity of the juice. It is also where up to 90 per cent of the flavones are found, along with a hefty helping of vitamin C. It may taste a tad bitter, but removing it could result in an eightfold decrease in the flavonoid content. Extracts of citrus peels have even been investigated as novel treatments for cancer, with one animal trial demonstrating that consuming them could reduce the volume of prostate tumours by as much as 94 per cent by killing cancer cells.

Segment membranes

Even in the flesh of the fruit, much of the bioactive compounds are found in tissues that may not always be consumed, and the thin membranes that separate each segment are a key example. These chewy fibres contain up to half of all the flavones found in the fruit flesh. If you peel these off or leave them behind by making conventionally squeezed juice from your oranges, you could be binning 50 per cent of the good stuff.

Flesh

Oranges may be a great source of vitamin C, but only 25 per cent of it is found in the juice. If you are going for juice, however, always pick unfiltered forms high in pulp, especially those made from comminuted orange juice, to reap the largest benefits.

HOW TO EAT ORANGE RIND, & LIKE IT

Orange skins might be packed full of the good stuff, but their intense bitterness can make eating them pretty hard going. Here are four recipes that use simple scientific tips and tricks to make them not just palatable, but downright delicious.

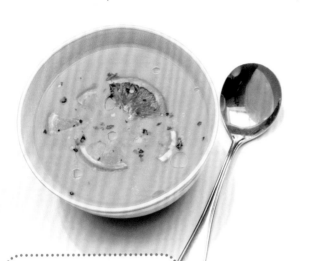

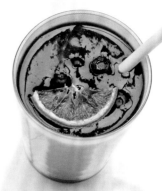

IN SMOOTHIES

When making your next smoothie, throw in ½ a whole orange for every 350ml glass you make. Sweet, creamy fruit like bananas, mangoes and papayas make the bitterness almost unnoticeable.

IN SOUP

I have found blending 1 whole orange with 1 litre of shop-bought carrot or pumpkin soup improves the flavour of the soup, adding only a hint of grown-up bitterness. Want to temper it? Simply add an indulgent swirl of cream when serving – the small amount of fat here acts as a solvent to dissolve the strong-tasting flavones and thus reduces the perception of bitterness.

IN ICE LOLLIES

Bitterness is less noticeable at lower temperatures, so freezing your smoothie to make an ice lolly is a great way to mask it. Unfortunately, it can also mask sweetness. This is easy to get over by adding a touch of stevia.

IN SQUASH

Put 2 roughly chopped whole oranges, 1 litre very cold water, a pinch of salt, the juice of 2 lemons, 1 tbsp double cream and 2 tbsp granulated stevia (baking blend) in a blender and blend together. Both the salt and the fat in the cream work to help mask any bitterness, plus you get a pleasant creamy mouthfeel. Serve immediately or store in the fridge for 2–3 days – just give it a good shake before serving.

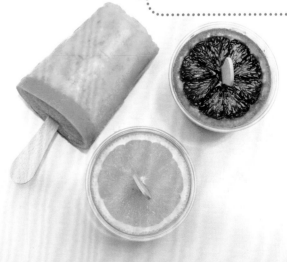

CITRUS CRISPS

I know these sound bonkers, but boy do they work! The idea came to me when I was reading a collection of studies that reported that oven-drying significantly enhanced the antioxidant power of citrus fruit. I whacked a couple of slices in the oven for a few hours to see what they tasted like and was astounded that the bitterness had been dramatically reduced, leaving behind a wafer-thin crisp with an intensely sugary, aromatic tang. These guys not only look and taste great, but could also contain between 60 and 70 per cent more polyphenols than fresh slices, which (in the words of one of the reports) could 'thus realize their outstanding potential for biomedical use'.

MAKES 50–60 SLICES
PREP TIME 5 MINUTES
COOK TIME 3 HOURS

....

6 MIXED ORANGES

PREHEAT the oven to 100°C/Gas Mark ¼.

SLICE the fruit very finely using a mandoline. (In theory you could slice these by hand, but you would need the skills of a surgeon to get them thin and even enough.)

SPREAD the slices out in a single layer on grill racks set over baking sheets.

BAKE for 3 hours, or until completely dehydrated and crisp, turning once halfway through the cooking time. Transfer to wire racks and leave to cool.

SERVE the crisps when cooled or store in airtight containers for up to 3 months.

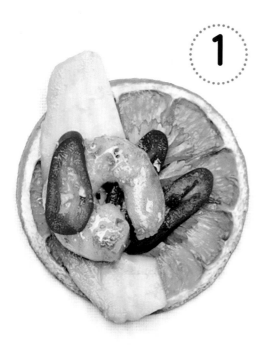

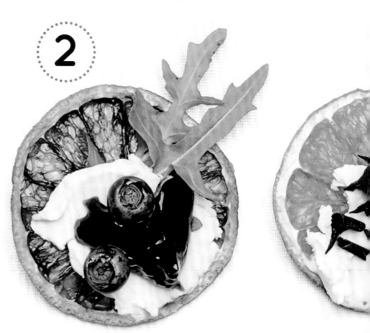

SUGGESTED TOPPINGS

(1) PRAWN & AVO

Pop a grilled **prawn** and a slice of **avocado** on an **orange crisp**, and decorate it with slices of **red chilli** and a **coriander leaf**.

(2) BLUEBERRY & GOATS' CHEESE

Smear a little **goats' cheese** on a **blood orange crisp** and top with a ¼ tsp of **Grape Jelly** (see page 147). Decorate with **blueberries** and **rocket leaves**.

(3) CHOCOLATE & ORANGE

Spread an **orange crisp** with 1 tsp of **ricotta cheese** and decorate it with a **mint leaf** and **dark chocolate** shavings.

(4) FIG & STILTON

Top an **orange crisp** with a thin sliver of **Stilton** and a slice of **fig** and decorate it with a few **pomegranate seeds** and a drizzle of **honey**.

(5) CITRUS & SEAFOOD

Spread some **soft cheese** on a **blood orange crisp** and top with some sliced **smoked salmon**, a **dill** frond and some **Pink Pickled Onions with Lime & Bay** (see page 64).

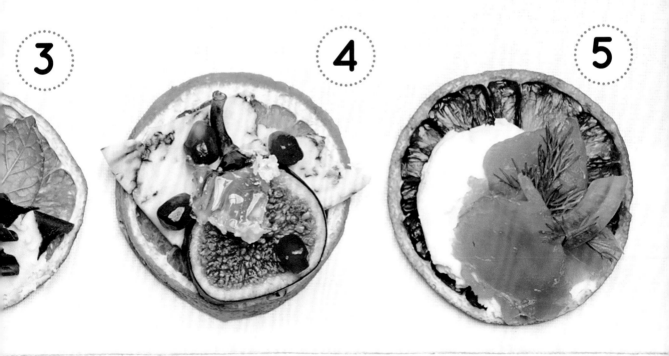

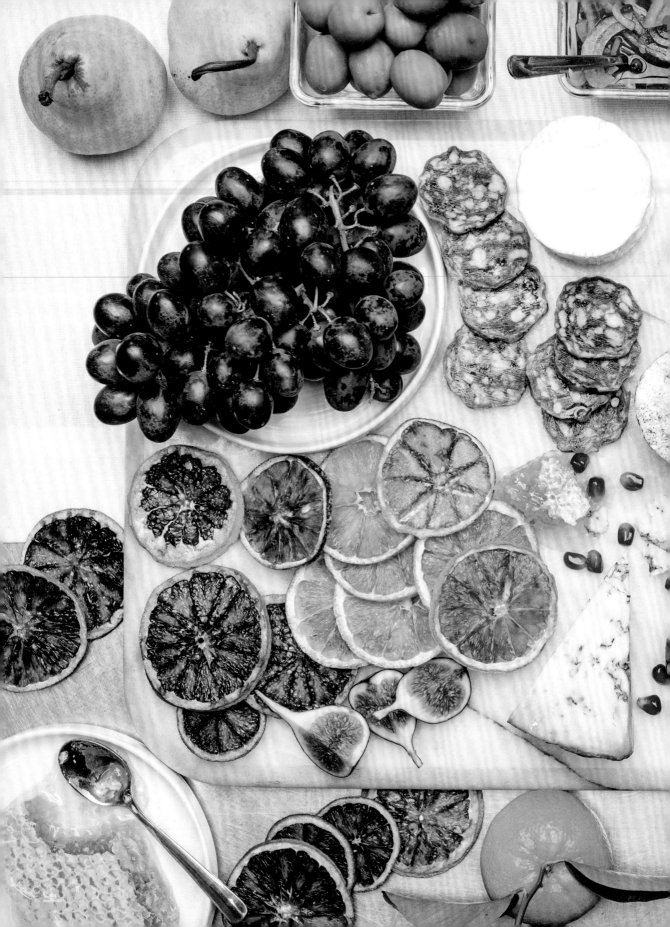

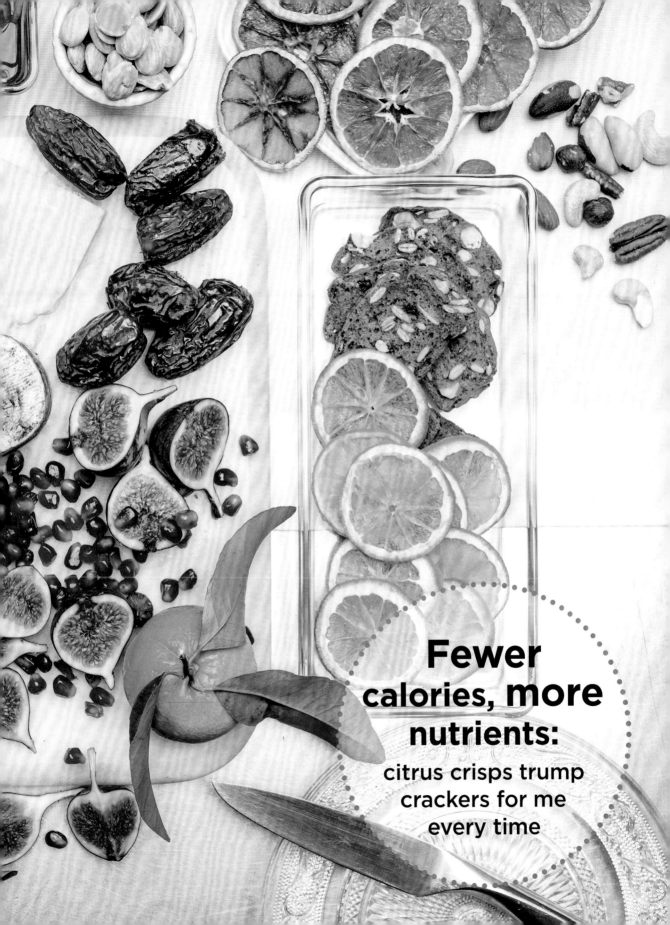

Fewer calories, more nutrients:

citrus crisps trump crackers for me every time

GRAPES

Irresistible sweetness, demonstrated health benefits and sold for less than half the price of other 'superfood' berries, few foods can boast quite as impressive a nutritional trifecta as grapes. Containing a unique cocktail of phytonutrients, which research has shown to potentially lower cholesterol, thin the blood, protect the body from free radical damage and even inhibit the proliferation of cancer cells (in test tubes, at least), grapes and their extracts have attracted a great deal of scientific interest. Here's the latest on what it has uncovered.

 ## CARDIO HEALTH

At least eight clinical studies have shown that consuming grape products may significantly improve the elasticity of blood vessels, thereby reducing the statistical risk of cardiovascular disease. This protective ability *could* be particularly beneficial to smokers, with one trial reporting that regular grape juice consumption helped prevent the immediate hardening of the arteries triggered by lighting up. Maintaining healthy arteries can have a direct impact on blood pressure and 'bad' LDL cholesterol, too, which are other risk factors for developing heart disease. Although results are mixed, there is emerging evidence to suggest that consuming grape products can even affect these, too. In one study at Korea's Kyung Hee University, for example, patients with stage 1 hypertension saw their blood pressure fall significantly after consuming a glass (about 350ml) of purple grape juice a day, reducing their status to pre-hypertension after just 8 weeks.

You may notice I haven't said 'grapes' but 'grape products' here. That's because the vast majority of studies have actually tested not the effect of the fruit itself, but grape *juice*. This might have a little something to do with the fact that many of these studies were funded by grape juice brands. Surprise!

 ## OXIDATIVE STRESS

After eating, particularly in the case of high-fat/high-carbohydrate meals, our bodies can enter a state known as postprandial oxidative stress. Here, the digestion process naturally generates potentially damaging free radicals, which can lower the body's own antioxidant defence and even lead to an immediate stiffening of the arteries by as much as 50 per cent. Not great. However, research at the Heart Center Research Program in the US found that consuming the phytonutrients contained in one large serving of purple grapes with a high-fat meal completely eliminated the significant hardening of the blood vessels that happened minutes after

exactly the same meal was eaten on its own. The fruit's apparent protective effect against free radicals has been noted by other studies, too, which showed that the levels of natural antioxidants in the bloodstream were maintained or even enhanced by scoffing grapes. I knew there was a reason cheese and grapes work so well together.

 ## BRAIN AGING

Research suggests that a daily dose of purple Concord grape juice may help slow age-related decline in memory and motor function in older adults after as little as 3 to 4 months, while boosting blood flow to the brain and even improving levels of concentration. But the benefits may not end there. A bunch of geeks at the University of Leeds decided to investigate whether the same juice could go further and improve the mental abilities of young, healthy people, too. Testing a group of working mums of pre-teen kids, researchers found that the women performed significantly better at driving tests designed to assess their spatial memory and reaction times after consuming a daily glass (about 350ml) of purple grape juice for 3 months. Moreover, the benefits persisted for more than a month after they ceased the consumption. Grapes make you a better driver, too, it seems.

 ## THE GREATEST GRAPES

But all grapes are not made equal. One of the key compounds thought to underpin the health benefits of eating grapes are the anthocyanin pigments, which give some varieties their rich purple (even black) colour. This is the same group of chemicals science suggests gives other crops like blueberries and purple carrots their intriguing biological effects and is almost totally absent in green types. Go for the very darkest you can and you will be rewarded with an astonishing nine times the antioxidants gram for gram, according to Cornell University. Here's a run-down of how they play out on the shelf.

MORE ANTIOXIDANTS

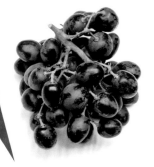

Sable Seedless
(purple-fleshed)

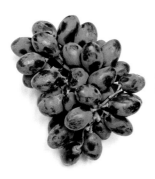

Autumn Royal
(green-fleshed)

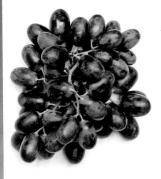

Crimson Seedless

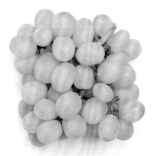

Thompson Seedless

Muscat de Alexandria

FEWER ANTIOXIDANTS

Black

Black grapes with both black skin and deep purple flesh are stained inside and out by anthocyanin pigments, giving them far and away the highest antioxidant activity. I particularly love Sable Seedless for its aromatic flavour and intense sweetness, 15 per cent higher in sugar than most other varieties.

Varieties with black skin but much lighter-coloured, green flesh tend to have fewer anthocyanins than those that are purple through and through. Bucking this trend however, the super-dark skin of Autumn Royal meant that it recently came out top in a study of red and black table grapes in the *Journal of Food Science*, containing more than twice the polyphenols of red grapes like Crimson Seedless and Red Globe.

Red

The rosy pink hue of red grapes comes from a light splash of the same pigments found in black grapes, which gives them the edge over green varieties. Picking a seeded variety and choosing bunches with the most intense colour will help you get that extra bit more benefit.

Green

Green grapes have the lowest polyphenols and antioxidant activity of all the major classes, which means you are likely to get far less nutritional bang for your buck. In one study on the effects of wine drinking, all products made out of black grapes (red wine, red wine extract and a mixed white and red wine extract) were shown to lower cholesterol levels, but white had no effect. The industry standard, Thompson Seedless, has a little as a third the antioxidant activity of some black table grapes, according to Cornell University.

OK, this is a heartbreaker for me. Muscat de Alexandria is easily one of my favourite varieties, with a syrupy sweetness and intense tropical lychee flavour. Sadly, it is about as low as they come in terms of polyphenols, with 40 per cent less than even Thompson Seedless. I hate it when the science isn't on my side!

🍳 GO FOR GREEN STEMS

Shipped from continent to continent in refrigerated storage, grapes experience a slow, but steady decline in their anthocyanin content. Despite giving the appearance of being freshly picked, some packets of supermarket grapes can be up to 4 weeks old and have lost close to half of their original colour and associated antioxidant benefits, at least according to Spain's Technical University of Cartagena. Interestingly, as the stems of grapes seem to deteriorate faster than the fruit itself, a dead giveaway is spotting bunches with plump, bright green stems. While the fruit may appear identical in packets whose stems have shrivelled to withered brown, these are often weeks older.

🍳 DITCH THE FRIDGE

There is an easy way to restore some of the original anthocyanin content of shop-bought grapes, according to the same Spanish team, and that is to simply take them out of the fridge. Removed from the chilled conditions of commercial storage and kept for 6 days at 15°C (the temperature of a cool room) the anthocyanin content was increased by as much as 20 per cent. So store them in the fruit bowl.

RAISINS

Dried to make raisins, the sweetness and nutrition of grapes are concentrated down to make a great high-energy snack on the go. In fact, two different studies have shown a serving of raisins (on average about 50g) to be as effective as commercial sports gels/chews at boosting athletic performance, despite being far cheaper, and with a concentrated dose of added phytonutrients.

While pretty much all the world's raisins (and sultanas for that matter) are made from a single green grape variety, Thompson Seedless, differences in how they are processed create a range of colours that are a telltale sign of their significant nutritional differences. Let me explain…

Sundried raisins

Made by spreading freshly harvested grapes out to dry naturally in the sun. Over several weeks a combination of heat and UV light triggers chemical reactions that break down a large proportion of the antioxidants in the fruit, creating an end product with comparatively low polyphenols. Natural is not always best.

Sultanas

Drying the same grapes in the shade shields the fruit from the most damaging effects of the sun, creating lighter-coloured raisins with more of their fresh flavour and nutrition intact. Different amounts of shade create different degrees of browning: the deeper the colour, the richer and more caramelized they will taste, but the lower antioxidant activity they are likely to have.

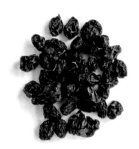
Sundried raisins

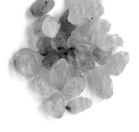
Golden raisins

Golden raisins

These guys are dried by being blasted by hot air, not shrivelling in the sun. This much faster process means the chemical reactions that degrade the fruit's natural polyphenols do not have time to take place. Adding sulphur dioxide to the fruit further helps preserve nutrition by blocking the action of the enzyme that causes this reaction. Brighter colour, fresher flavour and three times the antioxidants. Thank you science!

Currants, which are made by drying a small, intensely black grape cultivar from southern Greece, contain the **highest antioxidant levels of all**

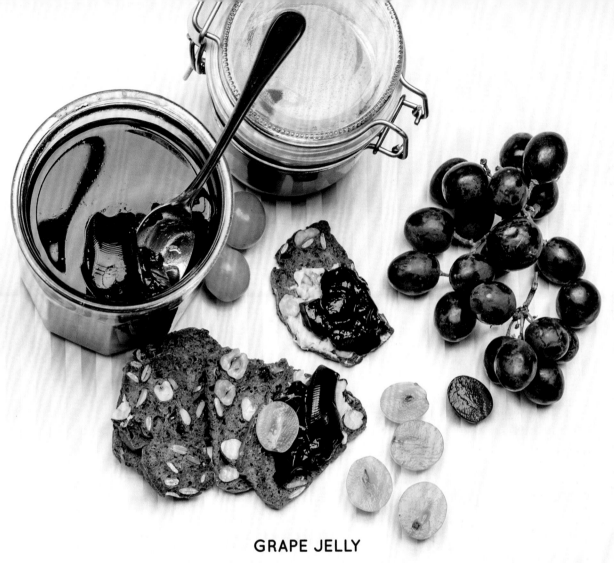

GRAPE JELLY

Grapes are naturally so intensely sweet they really don't need any added sugar to make a wonderful, healthy, US-style grape jelly. Instant good-mood food spread on wholegrain toast, dolloped on porridge and, of course, in a peanut butter and jelly sandwich.

MAKES 1 X 250ML JAR
PREP TIME 20 MINUTES
COOK TIME 5 MINUTES

....

2–4 SHEETS GELATINE (DEPENDING ON THE SET DESIRED)
500G DARK GRAPES
JUICE OF ½ LEMON

SOAK the gelatine in a bowl of cold water for 5–10 minutes, or until soft.

MEANWHILE, blitz the grapes and lemon juice in a food processor until as smooth as possible.

HEAT a third of the grape juice in a small saucepan until just below boiling point. Take off the heat, add the gelatine to the warmed juice and stir until dissolved. Pour the mixture back into the remaining grape juice and mix well.

POUR into a sterilized jar, immediately top with the lid and seal. Leave to set completely and store in the fridge for up to 2 weeks.

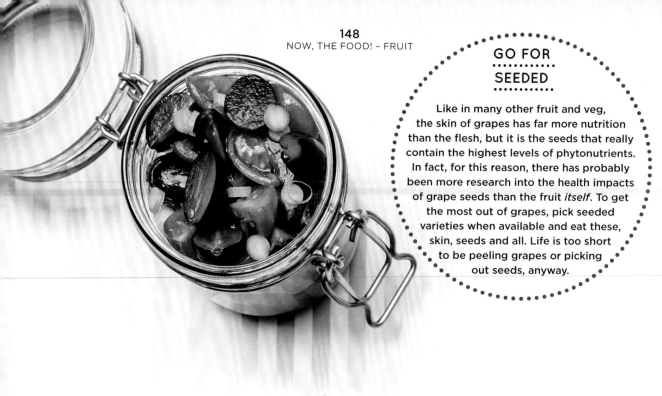

GO FOR
SEEDED

Like in many other fruit and veg, the skin of grapes has far more nutrition than the flesh, but it is the seeds that really contain the highest levels of phytonutrients. In fact, for this reason, there has probably been more research into the health impacts of grape seeds than the fruit *itself*. To get the most out of grapes, pick seeded varieties when available and eat these, skin, seeds and all. Life is too short to be peeling grapes or picking out seeds, anyway.

GRAPE SALSA

This classic sweet-sour combination works with cheese and chicken and meat dishes, just as a chutney would, except it's fresher, brighter and easier to make, without the ton of added sugar or hours of simmering. It is great with tacos, in sandwiches or just as a side salad.

MAKES ABOUT 500G

PREP TIME 15 MINUTES, PLUS STANDING

100G CHERRY TOMATOES, QUARTERED

100G DARK GRAPES, QUARTERED

3 SPRING ONIONS, CHOPPED

DRESSING

1 TSP CLEAR HONEY

2 TBSP CIDER VINEGAR

2 TBSP OLIVE OIL

1 TBSP FINELY CHOPPED TARRAGON

SALT AND PEPPER

PUT the tomatoes, grapes and spring onions in a non-reactive bowl and mix well.

WHISK the dressing ingredients together in another bowl.

POUR the dressing over the tomato mixture and mix through. Leave to stand for 1 hour before serving – this allows the flavours to combine. The salsa will keep, covered, in the fridge for up to 1 week.

NUTRITIONAL ANATOMY OF A GRAPE

You might have never known it, but this is where the polyphenols in grapes are hiding.

Seeds 87% ....

Skin 11% ....

Flesh 2% ....

GRAPE SORBET

Making sorbets without adding sugar is tricky. Without high concentrations of the sweet stuff, large ice crystals start to form, which can give the mix a distinctly crunchy, not smooth, texture. However, the naturally high sugar content in grapes prevents this from happening, and this three-ingredient sorbet is also quick and easy to make.

SERVES 4

PREP TIME 10 MINUTES, PLUS FREEZING

300G DARK GRAPES, PICKED OFF THE STALKS AND FROZEN, PLUS EXTRA TO SERVE

JUICE OF ½ LEMON

PINCH OF SALT

BLITZ the frozen grapes with the lemon juice and salt in a food processor, then transfer to a large plastic tub or tray, cover and freeze for at least 30 minutes or until nearly solid.

SCOOP the sorbet into serving bowls and serve with fresh grapes.

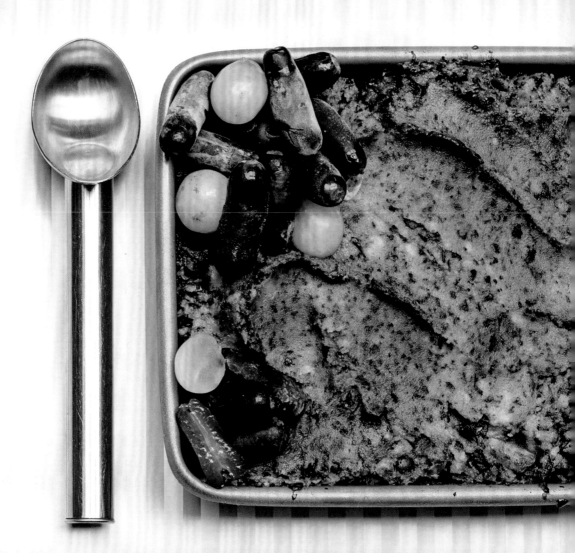

MANGOES

Silky smooth, intensely sweet and with an aroma second to none, to me mangoes are the king of all fruit. And that is before we get on to their growing list of intriguing potential health benefits. Here's the latest science has to say.

♡ A SUPERIOR SOURCE OF VITAMIN A

With your full recommended daily dose of vitamin C and more than half the vitamin A you need in every 150g, mangoes were always known to be an excellent source of essential nutrients. However, now some intriguing new research suggests that in the vitamin A stakes they may be even better than previously thought. Unlike in veg such as carrots and tomatoes, the carotenes in mangoes (which our bodies convert to vitamin A) are not tightly bound to solid crystals but found sloshing about in liquid form in the cells of the fruit. This makes them far easier to absorb. Twenty times more, in fact, than those in carrots and three times more than tomatoes, according to a team at Germany's University of Hohenheim.

♡ 'MAGIC' MANGIFERIN?

Mangoes are also a unique dietary source of a natural polyphenol. Found nowhere else in nature, some initial studies suggest, alongside the fruit's rich fibre content, this novel compound – mangiferin – may have some pretty intriguing effects on blood sugar and fat levels. One pilot study at Oklahoma State University reported that eating the equivalent of half a mango a day for 12 weeks could significantly limit sugar absorption and insulin sensitivity in a small group of obese men and women. Theoretically, over the long term this might lower diabetes risk and even help control appetite, although in the short duration of the trial none of the subjects actually lost weight. These findings, however, add to those of a larger clinical trial that reported that people taking a mangiferin supplement had lower levels of triglycerides, improved insulin resistance and even boosted 'good' HDL cholesterol levels. Several recent animal studies also suggest that mangiferin supplementation, as well as just eating mangoes, could lower blood sugar levels and reduce weight gain.

Intriguing? Yes. Conclusive? Well, not yet at least. But in the meantime, for a simple way to send the amount of mangiferin in your mangoes skyrocketing, as if by magic, see 'Eat Them Skin & All' on page 151.

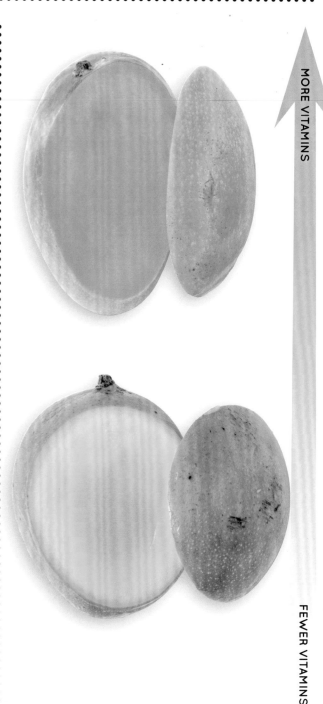

MORE VITAMINS

FEWER VITAMINS

PICK THE YELLOW ONES

The easiest way to boost the nutritional value of your mangoes is to simply pick the right variety. As there's only a few available this is super-easy to do, yet could give you several times more of the good stuff.

Long & yellow

These varieties originate in Southeast Asia, are the most popular ones in Asian grocery stores and are becoming increasingly common in the larger supermarkets. This group, perhaps confusingly, also includes the Mexican variety Ataulfo, which is very popular in the United States and was originally introduced by the Spanish from the Philippines in the 1700s. Why bother making the effort? Well, according to the United States Department of Agriculture, varieties like this consistently contain up to five times the vitamins A and C of the rock-hard green ones – in fact, more than any other varieties it tested.

You can see the difference in vitamin A potential just by looking at them, as the carotene pigments our bodies use to manufacture vitamin A dye the flesh a deep orange hue. Plus, as many of the flavour compounds that give mangoes their irresistible aroma come from a breakdown of carotenes, the brighter the flesh the better they taste. These mangoes also have a silkier, pudding-like texture, without those stringy fibres that get stuck in your teeth. I know I am biased, but when it comes to mangoes, the Asian ones really are always the best.

Round & green

Sadly, the mangoes most commonly sold in my local supermarkets are the round, green ones like Kent and Tommy Atkins. Bred in the USA in the 1920s for their superior size, shelf life and disease resistance, they dominate the European and North American markets, but have just a fraction of the nutrients, and in my opinion flavour, of others out there. Sidestep these, if you can.

Yellow-skinned mangoes can contain **5X MORE** vitamins C and A than round and **green mangoes**

EAT THEM SKIN & ALL

Mango peel contains an astonishing 400 times the mangiferin than the fruit itself and is – perhaps surprisingly to some people – totally edible. This is particularly true for the yellow, Asian-type mangoes, which, besides having higher nutritional value, tend to have much, much thinner skins and are traditionally eaten unpeeled. Yet another reason to pick these tasty varieties over the nutritionally inferior round, green type. Therefore, simply not peeling your fruit before you slice it into a fruit salad, chuck it in a smoothie or make my delicious Mango & Saffron Pudding (see page 152) can give you up to 100 times the mangiferin per serving, not to mention fibre and loads more antioxidant carotenes too. More nutrition for less work, and I promise with the yellow variety you will barely notice.

Now here's the catch. A small minority of people are allergic to a compound called urushiol (pronounced u-roo-shee-ol) that is found in the resin of mango trees, including in the fruit peel. This is the sticky, clear liquid you often find dripping from the cut stem where the mango was once attached to the tree, and is chemically similar to that found in poison ivy and poison oak (two relatives of mango trees), albeit at much lower doses. Known as 'mango rash' in Hawaii, uncommon symptoms include irritation and dermatitis. If you have a strong sensitivity to either of these plants, or have experienced reactions after eating unripe mangoes – think Thai green mango salad – or mango chutney (both of which contain higher doses of urushiol than ripe fruit), you should avoid eating mango peel.

TROPICAL FRUIT LOVE
TROPICAL TEMPERATURES

Pop your mango on the work surface rather than in the fridge for a few days and you can get loads more carotenes and even sweeter fruit, according to the *Journal of the Science of Food and Agriculture*. As fruit ripens between about 22°C and 32°C (the temperature of your average warm kitchen) it starts churning out up to twice the carotenes than those stored at 12–17°C or lower.

The same treatment also causes the acid content of the fruit to plummet up to 80 per cent compared to those kept in the fridge, making them taste far sweeter despite containing the same amount of sugar. Far more flavour and nutrition for simply not bothering to open the fridge? I think that's a fair deal.

MANGO & SAFFRON PUDDING

In my research on mangoes I found all sorts of weird and wonderful studies. Everything from a report from the University of Queensland, which found that puréeing mango fruit caused its betacarotenes to be twice as well absorbed (good news for smoothie lovers), to a trial in the *Journal of Food Science and Technology* that suggested the proteins in milk could have a similar effect when consumed with carotenes. Just like carrots and tomatoes, adding a little fat to mangoes also helped significantly boost their potential vitamin A. What if I could do this all in one recipe? Well, here it is: a smooth, sweet mango pudding, like that of dim sum dreams, that swaps the added sugar for a boatload more potential nutrition.

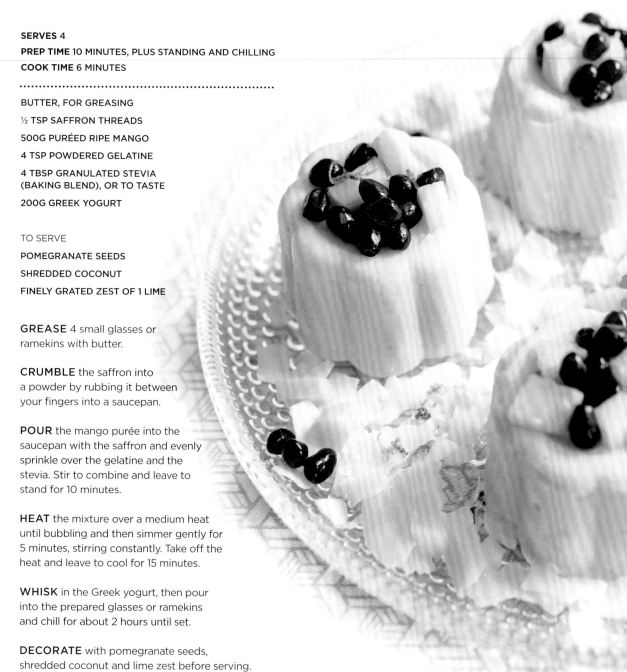

SERVES 4
PREP TIME 10 MINUTES, PLUS STANDING AND CHILLING
COOK TIME 6 MINUTES

···

BUTTER, FOR GREASING

½ TSP SAFFRON THREADS

500G PURÉED RIPE MANGO

4 TSP POWDERED GELATINE

4 TBSP GRANULATED STEVIA (BAKING BLEND), OR TO TASTE

200G GREEK YOGURT

TO SERVE

POMEGRANATE SEEDS

SHREDDED COCONUT

FINELY GRATED ZEST OF 1 LIME

GREASE 4 small glasses or ramekins with butter.

CRUMBLE the saffron into a powder by rubbing it between your fingers into a saucepan.

POUR the mango purée into the saucepan with the saffron and evenly sprinkle over the gelatine and the stevia. Stir to combine and leave to stand for 10 minutes.

HEAT the mixture over a medium heat until bubbling and then simmer gently for 5 minutes, stirring constantly. Take off the heat and leave to cool for 15 minutes.

WHISK in the Greek yogurt, then pour into the prepared glasses or ramekins and chill for about 2 hours until set.

DECORATE with pomegranate seeds, shredded coconut and lime zest before serving.

CHERRIES

If I had to pick just one fruit to live off forever, it would have to be the deep, dark deliciousness of the cherry. Just as well then that, on top of loads of vitamins, minerals and fibre, early research is also beginning to reveal some fascinating effects that the phytonutrients they contain may have on our bodies. Here's a peek at what we know so far.

 ## EXERCISE RECOVERY

Cherries contain a heady cocktail of anti-inflammatory compounds. So much so that research suggests they may possess a similar level of efficacy to non-steroidal anti-inflammatory drugs like aspirin. This is intriguing to researchers because despite being very effective, these conventional medications can often have undesirable side-effects, particularly when used at high doses over the long term. From causing damage to the stomach lining to, in extreme cases, salicylism (a toxic build-up of aspirin in the body for which there is no antidote), these side effects can be pretty nasty indeed.

Wouldn't it be interesting, therefore, if cherries could be used as a tasty way to alleviate pain and inflammation, such as that induced by strenuous exercise, with potentially fewer side-effects? A team of researchers at Northumbria University thought so, finding this so interesting, in fact, that they set up a small clinical trial. They gave a bunch of runners daily servings of either cherry juice or artificially flavoured cherry cordial with similar appearance, caloric content and taste (but no phytonutrients) in the 5 days leading up to a marathon. The cherry drinkers not only saw their post-run strength recover significantly faster, but also their levels of pain and inflammation were reduced. Blood tests also revealed elevated antioxidant levels, causing the researchers to conclude that 'cherry juice appears to provide a viable means to aid recovery following strenuous exercise'.

Similar results of faster recovery times, reduced pain and improved strength have been found by other teams looking at comparable doses of cherry juice in runners, cyclists and gym goers. How much stronger are we talking? Juice-drinking college students made to do bicep curls until exhaustion set in saw only a 4 per cent loss of strength in one trial by the University of Vermont compared to a whopping 22 per cent loss in the control group, an impressive fivefold difference. The scientists, however, sound like a bunch of sadists.

 ## ARTHRITIS

Reducing inflammation is essentially what drugs used to treat arthritis do, so drinking cherry juice could theoretically also benefit patients with gout, one of the most common arthritic conditions. In a small pilot study published in the *Journal of Arthritis*, consuming 2 tablespoons of cherry juice concentrate a day was found to be significantly more effective than a placebo drink at reducing the incidence of gout attacks – by as much as 60 per cent, in fact. More than half the patients in the cherry juice group who were already on conventional anti-inflammatory drugs found that their symptoms improved so much they were even able to discontinue their medication after 2 months of juice drinking, compared to none in the placebo group. This was, however, just a single, tiny study, using a grand total of 14 patients (only 9 of whom actually consumed cherry juice). But while we wait for further clinical studies to add more context to these findings, they do echo a wider body of evidence that suggests cherry juice consumption can have significant anti-inflammatory effects with no reported side-effects. The stuff is hardly a chore to drink either.

 ## RESTFUL SLEEP

Here's the weird thing with science – sometimes when you investigate one thing you make other equally exciting discoveries along the way. In the aforementioned University of Vermont exercise study, some participants anecdotally reported they were sleeping better, a phenomenon also mentioned by athletes taking the juice as a sports supplement. This piqued the interest of the lab geeks because, in addition to their anti-inflammatory chemicals, cherries are also known to contain a compound called melatonin, a hormone that regulates sleep patterns in humans. The amount our brains produce tends to decrease as we age, which may explain why insomnia rates are higher in older people, and it was already known that taking synthetic melatonin in pill form could improve sleep. Putting two and two together, a team of US researchers decided to investigate this and indeed found giving older insomniacs a dose of cherry juice resulted in not only increased levels of melatonin in their blood, but also modest but significant improvement in sleep quality. Although the total length of sleep time wasn't affected much, the subjects would often fall asleep faster and wake up less frequently in the night. The curious thing is, this study didn't actually administer pure cherry juice, but a proprietary blend watered down with 50 per cent apple juice.

When the experiment was repeated in a study published by the *European Journal of Nutrition* using full-strength cherry juice, with twice the cherry content of the cherry/apple blend, study participants experienced not only improved sleep quality but also an extra 34 minutes of sleep on average. These results were seen after just 7 days of drinking two 250ml glasses of cherry juice per day. A third study at the Louisiana State University even reported up to 85 minutes of increased sleep using the same dosage of full-strength juice, but using a much smaller group of participants. Add a natural sleep hormone to calming anti-inflammatories and you just might have a recipe for better sleep with a cherry on top.

🧺 WHICH ONES WORK BEST?

OK, I'll admit I have been a bit naughty so far – I have lumped all sorts of cherries together as a single entity. However – perhaps more than for any other fruit – there is a really clear indication that one type of cherry is not only more nutrient dense, but also has greater evidence of health benefits. Here is where I come clean.

ORGANIZZZ

Melatonin might help you nod off quicker, but what is a human brain hormone doing in plants? Well, the answer is we still don't know. In fact, it was only discovered in plants in 1995. As it has antioxidant effects and is produced more by plants under stress, we suspect it may have something to do with protection from UV radiation, drought or disease, or maybe all three.

As organically grown crops tend to have more pest damage and therefore often contain high concentrations of defence chemicals, this *might* suggest that organic sour cherries could contain more melatonin. However, in the absence of a trial, we will just have to wait and see!

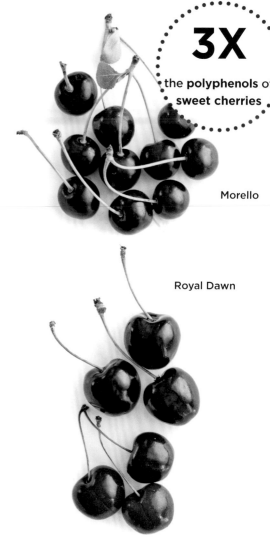

3X the **polyphenols** of **sweet cherries**

Morello

Royal Dawn

Penny

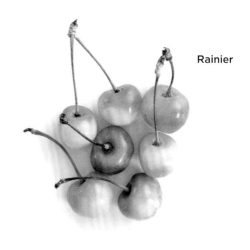

Rainier

Sour cherries

These poor guys haven't had it easy over the last 50 years. In my native UK, for example, there were dozens of varieties of sour cherries grown commercially before the Second World War. Now you would be lucky to find more than one. This isn't just a shame for our taste buds, but potentially for our health, too, as they contain significantly more phytonutrients. As much as triple the polyphenols – in particular, the red and purple anthocyanin pigments – as the regular sweet types, according to the *Journal of Agricultural and Food Chemistry*.

Not to mention also being higher in a whole alphabet soup of vitamins, including A, B, C, E and K. This is pretty crucial as scientists believe it is these polyphenols that explain the anti-inflammatory properties of cherries. This was neatly reflected in the study above, which also found that the cherry extracts with the strongest protective effect on brain cells in test tubes were those with the highest polyphenol content. While tracking down the fresh fruit can be tricky, sour cherries (sometimes called 'tart cherries') are extremely widely sold in juice form, not to mention becoming increasingly common in the frozen section of supermarkets. And the best news is that research suggests that they retain their health benefits even after processing. In fact, all the trials showing intriguing benefits have been done exclusively on the juice of the sour kind.

Sweet cherries

But who wants to eat sour cherries, when you can have sweet ones? I have news for you. 'Sour' cherries are so named because they contain more acid, but they often contain just as much if not more sugar, which often makes them pretty sweet, too. A fully ripe Morello will knock the socks off any watery so-called 'sweet' supermarket staple any day of the week. As a large part of the polyphenols in cherries comes from their anthocyanin pigments, picking the black varieties over the paler reds will instantly give you as much as 50 per cent more of the good stuff.

Yellow cherries

These yellow and pink-blushed beauties have only recently started appearing at my local supermarket, sold at a premium price – presumably for their visual novelty? Although they taste just like the regular kind, studies show these paler cousins can have as little as 1 per cent of the anthocyanins of the equally sweet black types. Same flavour, higher price, 99 per cent less potential benefit? I know which one I'd pick.

WORRIED ABOUT THE SUGAR?

The doses of cherry juice used in the trials that suggest their numerous health benefits are not ridiculous – about two small glasses (500ml) a day. This is, however, about three times the amount of fruit juice many official guidelines, like those of Public Health England, now recommend. As juicing removes the healthy fibre from the fruit, which normally blunts its impact on blood sugar, drinking large amounts of juice is not considered preferable to consuming the whole food.

Fortunately, there are some things you can do about this, such as 'replacing' some of the lost fibre by stirring a spoonful of chia or flaxseed into your glass of cherry juice. If you aren't a fan of the texture, whack the lot in a blender. You can even add pieces of whole fruit, too, which will further increase the fibre and phytonutrient content, making a tasty smoothie. Of course, simply drinking any of these variations with a meal, instead of on its own, will have a similar effect in quelling the impact of the sugar.

Finally, it is worth noting that the polyphenols found in cherries, as with several berry species, may actually help lessen the impact of the sugar they contain on blood glucose in the first place, so in the context of other treats (think sweets, cakes and biscuits) a cherry smoothie really isn't the worst option. Bottoms up!

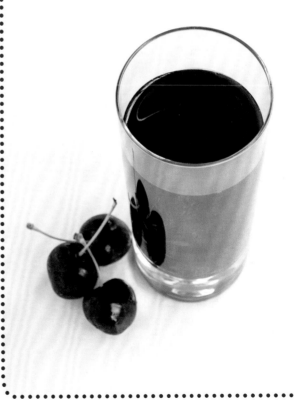

CHERRY COMPOTE

Glossy red, sweet deliciousness – every year I wait for sour cherry season with bated breath to make this stuff. It freezes wonderfully, too, so I make a massive batch to freeze in sealable freezer bags to last me all year.

MAKES 300G

PREP TIME 5 MINUTES

COOK TIME 3 MINUTES

....

300G MORELLO CHERRIES, PITTED

1 TBSP ARROWROOT OR CORNFLOUR

1 TSP MIXED SPICE

1 TBSP GRANULATED STEVIA (BAKING BLEND)

FINELY GRATED ZEST AND JUICE OF 1 LEMON

PLACE all the ingredients in a microwaveable bowl and stir to combine.

COOK in a microwave on high for 3 minutes, stirring halfway through the cooking time. Leave to cool slightly before serving.

STORE the compote in the fridge for up to 1 week.

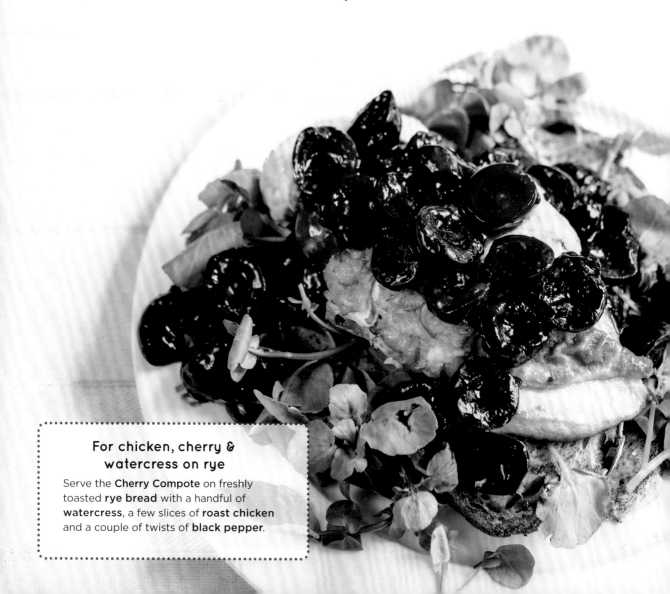

For chicken, cherry & watercress on rye

Serve the **Cherry Compote** on freshly toasted **rye bread** with a handful of **watercress**, a few slices of **roast chicken** and a couple of twists of **black pepper**.

CHICKPEA & BROWN SUGAR PANCAKES WITH CHERRY COMPOTE

The breakfast of kings, these pancakes made with protein-packed chickpea flour have an incredible moreish texture and will keep you fuller for longer. A match made in cherry-chickpea heaven.

SERVES 2
PREP TIME 10 MINUTES
COOK TIME 10 MINUTES

150G CHICKPEA FLOUR
2 EGGS
150G CANNED SWEETCORN KERNELS, RINSED AND DRAINED
1 TBSP DEMERARA SUGAR
1 TSP MIXED SPICE
FINELY GRATED ZEST AND JUICE OF 1 ORANGE
1 TSP VANILLA ESSENCE
½ TSP BAKING POWDER
LARGE PINCH OF SALT
1 TBSP MELTED BUTTER, PLUS EXTRA FOR GREASING

TO SERVE
CHERRY COMPOTE (SEE PAGE 156)
FRESH FRUIT

PUT all the ingredients in a food processor and blitz until you have a smooth batter.

GREASE a large frying pan with butter and heat until hot, then pour spoonfuls of the chunky batter into the pan to make small pancakes the size of a CD. Cook for about 1 minute on each side until golden and cooked through. Remove from the pan and keep warm in a low oven until all the pancakes are made.

SLATHER the compote over a towering stack of pancakes and serve with fresh fruit

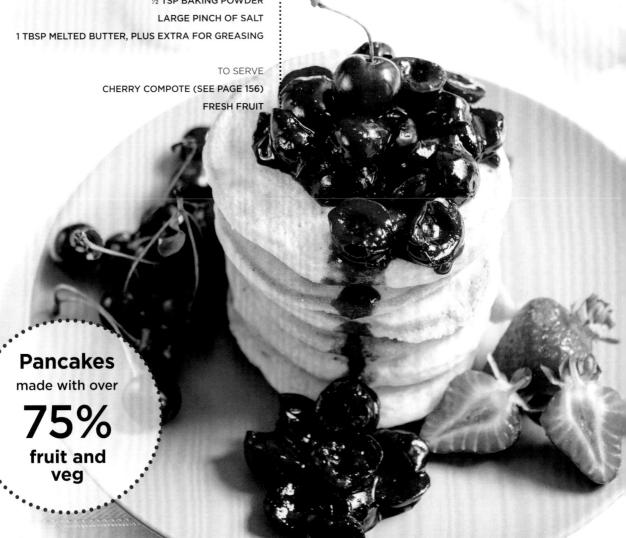

Pancakes made with over **75%** fruit and veg

PINEAPPLES

New breeding work on pineapples has made them sweeter and tastier, with a massive amount more nutrition. If you only know these guys through tasteless canned rings, I implore you to give them another go. Your health might just thank you for it!

 IMMUNE BOOST?

Dishing up your entire recommended daily dose of vitamin C per 150g serving, not to mention a whole bunch of other essential vitamins and minerals like vitamin B6, folate and copper, pineapples are not lacking in nutritional boasts. As some evidence from animal studies suggests that these exact nutrients are important for healthy immune function, could tucking into more pineapple ward off colds?

In one small trial, published in the *Journal of Nutrition and Metabolism,* adding a few generous servings of canned pineapple to schoolchildren's diets (a population segment at higher risk of catching respiratory infections) could not only slash their rates of everyday infections like colds and flu by 50 per cent, but also significantly shorten the duration of the illness. Sounds amazing!

However, it's important to point out that the study was carried out in the Philippines and a significant proportion of these kids were sadly reported by the researchers to have existing nutrient deficiencies, so they may have benefitted more from the added fruit than otherwise healthy children. Why canned pineapple? Well, the study was funded by a canned pineapple manufacturer (no surprise there) so fresh fruit may work even better.

 CALMING INFLAMMATION?

Uniquely, fresh pineapples also contain an enzyme called bromelain, which has shown early promise in test-tube and animal studies for reducing inflammation and pain and even inhibiting the growth of cancer cells. Eating the fruit has therefore been widely recommended in fitness mags as an essential pre/post-workout snack to supposedly help your body recover from the stresses and strains of physical exertion. It is even routinely claimed to help inflammatory diseases such as arthritis and IBS for the same reason.

Evidence from human trials, however, is currently limited and the results often conflicting. What makes a like-for-like comparison even trickier is that most trials have not fed people actual pineapples, but purified bromelain. This extract isn't derived from the fruit itself but from the stem and leaves of pineapple plants, and is chemically distinct from the type of bromelain found in the fruit. These studies have generally also tested doses *far* higher than the amount you could be realistically expected to eat in fresh fruit (we are talking kilo after kilo). So the jury is still *very* much out on whether these claims stack up.

 DIGESTIVE HEALTH

However, there is one property about bromelain that has excellent evidence: its ability to digest protein, even in the doses found naturally in fresh fruit. This makes raw pineapples a very effective meat tenderizer and therefore may be beneficial for people who are prone to indigestion after protein-heavy meals, in theory. As bromelain is capable of withstanding stomach acid, it may be effective not only as a marinade prior to cooking, but also eaten in conjunction with meat dishes too. It does have to be *raw* pineapple though, as the all-important bromelian gets destroyed by heat (that includes pineapple in cans and shop-bought juice). Just as well then that pineapple salsa goes with pretty much everything.

DITCH THE
JUICE

Not only does juicing remove healthful fibre, causing the sugar content per serving to soar, but most of the carotenes in pineapple are bound to this fibre, meaning that juice has 80 per cent fewer of these essential antioxidants than fresh fruit.

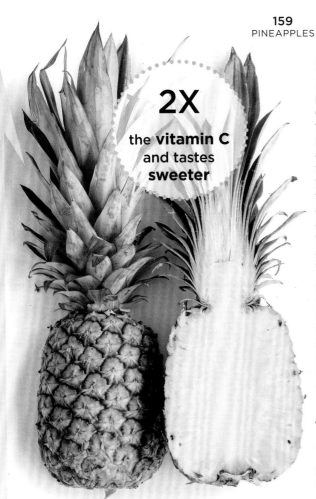

MORE VITAMINS

2X

the **vitamin C** and tastes **sweeter**

FEWER VITAMINS

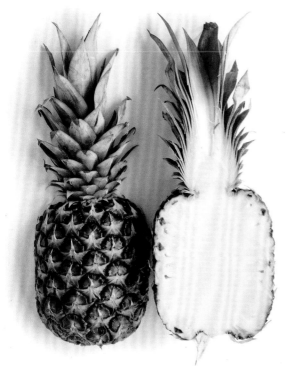

Supersweets

Introduced in the 1990s, not only are 'supersweet' pineapples significantly sweeter tasting, they also come with supercharged nutrition. According to the University of Hawaii, compared to traditional pineapples we are talking twice the vitamin C and nearly three times the antioxidant carotenes, which coincidentally also give them a lovely, deep yellow colour. But should we really be breeding things to make them sweeter? What about all the extra sugar? Well, surprisingly, the supersweets actually contain the same amount of sugar as the traditional variety but half the mouth-puckering acid, which makes their existing sweetness come to the fore.

Sold under a range of glossy marketing names, often including 'gold' or 'Hawaii', these supersweets are all actually a single variety with the rather unglamorous official title of MD2 (although you will never see this on the packaging). Sadly, plant breeders are not known for their romantic side). Whatever the name, the word 'supersweet' on the label is a dead giveaway.

Traditional

Supersweets are quickly beginning to replace the single traditional cultivar that once had a virtual monopoly on global pineapple production. Called Smooth Cayenne – its leaves are free of spines, which makes for easier harvesting – this variety was first bred by indigenous South Americans and can date its origins right back to precolonial times. Yet its sharp flavour meant the vast majority of pineapple was eaten canned until as recently as 20 years ago, often with a hefty dose of added sugar. That was until the nutritionally enhanced supersweets caused a global boom in sales of pineapples tasty enough to be eaten fresh – yet more evidence to show that when it comes to food, 'heritage' or 'heirloom' varieties don't necessarily go hand in hand with better flavour or nutrition.

Both the sugar and nutrient levels in pineapples peak just before they reach full maturity when their skins are three-quarters yellow, as seen in the photo here. So impatient pineapple lovers don't need to leave them any longer.

PINEAPPLE ACHAR

This is a nifty way to pack even more fruit and veg on your plate at your next barbecue. It works wonderfully as either a meat-tenderizing marinade or a simple salsa. Lean, grilled chicken, tangy pineapple and creamy peanut sauce make an irresistible trifecta on a hot summer day.

MAKES 6–8 SKEWERS

PREP TIME 25 MINUTES, PLUS MARINATING

COOK TIME 8 MINUTES

½ PINEAPPLE, SKIN REMOVED, CORED AND FINELY DICED

½ RED ONION, THINLY SLICED

½ CUCUMBER, FINELY DICED

1 RED CHILLI, THINLY SLICED

100ML CIDER VINEGAR

1 TBSP CRUSHED GARLIC

1 TBSP PEELED AND MINCED FRESH ROOT GINGER

1 TBSP CASTER SUGAR

JUICE OF 1 LIME

½ TSP SALT

COMBINE all the achar ingredients together in a non-reactive bowl, cover and leave to macerate in the fridge for at least 30 minutes.

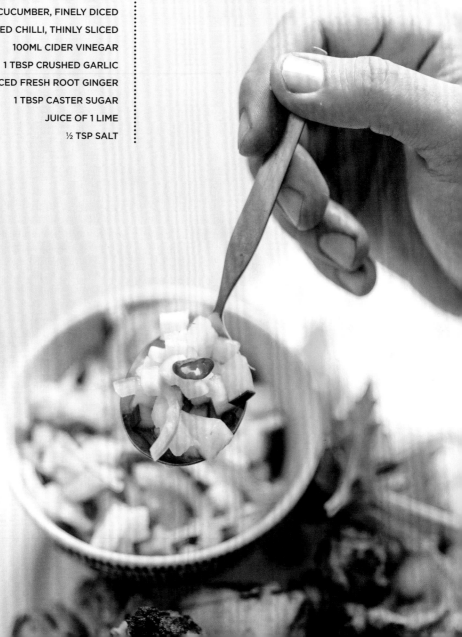

PLUMS & PEACHES

When it comes to the wonderful world of 'superfood' claims, peaches and plums rarely get a mention. To me this has always been surprising, as even a cursory look at nutritional tables will show the lowly plum, for example, has a comparable level of most essential vitamins and minerals to celebrated 'superfood' blueberries, not to mention similar levels of polyphenols and antioxidant activity. I guess plum growers haven't been quite as quick to get the PR machine behind them? But that just means you get plenty of the good stuff without the trendy 'clean-eating' price tag. Here are my top tips for getting the very best out of these two delicious fruits.

BONE BOOSTING?

The vast bulk of the research into the health benefits of these fruit has centred on plums, which have roughly twice the polyphenols of peaches. Chief among the research are a range of test-tube, animal and human studies that suggest the phytonutrients in plums may help slow (and even reverse) the progression of osteoporosis. Let me explain...

Our bones contain two types of cells: osteo*blasts*, which help build a strong matrix of dense bone tissue using the calcium in our diets, and osteo*clasts*, which break down ageing bone by firing destructive chemicals called free radicals at it so it can be replaced by the new. An imbalance of this activity is associated with age-related bone loss, as old bone is degraded faster than it can be replaced. Diets rich in antioxidants such as polyphenols, however, are thought to help redress this balance, mopping up the excess free radicals to create stronger bone tissue. Snacking on 10–12 dried plums a day for 3 months was enough to significantly increase bone density in postmenopausal women, according to Oklahoma State University, with a trial at the University of Florida suggesting very similar results. But polyphenols can be found in all sorts of fruit, so are plums in any way special? Well, out of five different dried polyphenol-rich fruit, including apples, apricots, grapes and mangoes, only dried plums were found to have this bone-protecting property in animal tests. This may be because on top of their rich polyphenol content, plums are also a good source of vitamin K, boron, manganese, copper and potassium, all of which are thought to play a role in bone health. Sounds like a pretty potent cocktail! But the promise doesn't end there – dried plums have also been associated with a lowered 'bad' LDL cholesterol level in some (but not all) trials, and even improved mental function in studies using ageing lab mice. Much more research is needed, but this all points to the idea that plums can be one of the healthiest snacks about.

WHY PRUNES KEEP YOU REGULAR

It might seem surprising that anyone needed to conduct a clinical trial to prove this, but at least three studies appear to have done just that. Yes, eating prunes does apparently help keep you regular. In fact, in two of these trials they appeared to work as well if not better than the active ingredient in the standard over-the-counter treatment, Metamucil, in providing 'immediate relief' – leading researchers of one study to conclude that being 'safe, palatable and more effective...[they] should be considered a first line of therapy'. According to these studies, a single dose of 7–8 prunes is apparently all you need to do the trick.

Yet according to Johns Hopkins School of Public Health in the USA, we still don't know what exactly it is in prunes that is responsible for this effect. They do contain plenty of fibre, but so do other foods that don't have the same properties. They also contain sorbitol, a sweet-tasting sugar alcohol that draws water into the digestive tract and may feed friendly gut bacteria, which is almost certainly adding to it. Finally, they contain polyphenols that have known anti-inflammatory effects, which may be playing a role, too. A three-way combination therapy, it seems.

Plums have

2x

the **polyphenols** of **peaches**

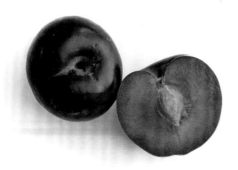

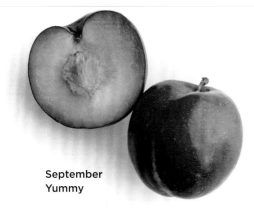

Queen Garnet

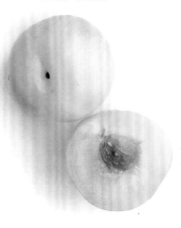

September
Yummy

⏛ PLUMS

On average, plums contain roughly twice the polyphenols of peaches; however, they vary incredibly widely between cultivars, with some possessing many times the phytonutrients of others. Luckily for those of us who don't carry lab equipment to the supermarket with us, there is a simple giveaway to the ones with the highest levels of polyphenols on the shelves: their colour.

Red & purple

These varieties have a similar basic make-up to yellow and green fruit in terms of vitamins and minerals, but come with the bonus of heart-healthy anthocyanin pigments that dye their skin (and often flesh) a deeper, darker hue. The blacker they are, the more they are likely to contain, according to the United States Department of Agriculture, making them a superior choice to yellow and green types in the antioxidant stakes.

Yellow & green

These have the lowest amount of polyphenols – on average, levels are 25 per cent lower than the red types, according to Venezuela's Simón Bolívar University. They do contain some antioxidant betacarotene, which gives them their pretty colour – however, this is present in roughly equal amounts in all plum varieties, it's just often masked by dark red and purple pigments in the darker, more nutrient-dense forms.

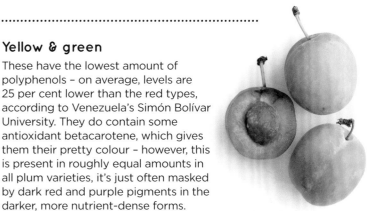

Reine Claude

Shiro

ALL HAIL QUEEN GARNET

Upping the levels of phytonutrients in crops has been one of the key focuses of modern breeding. One of the most recent commercial successes is a new Aussie hybrid, Queen Garnet. Developed with funding from the Queensland government, she boasts a near-black interior created by more than twice the anthocyanins of normal plums and very early research has suggested this could have positive effects on some measures of heart-disease risk factors in humans. When I say 'early', one of these trials had a grand total of two, yes two, participants – but with great flavour, stunning colour and measurably more of the good stuff, I'd happily pick the queen over her paler plum cousins when in season.

THE SMALLER,
THE BETTER

Like many fruit, the polyphenols and antioxidant activity in plums are heavily concentrated in the skin. In some paler-fleshed varieties, this thin layer can contain more than seven times that of the flesh within, meaning the smaller-fruited forms, which contain proportionately more skin, gram for gram, will generally be a more nutrient-rich choice. I am looking at you, damsons and mirabelles.

HIGHEST ANTIOXIDANTS

9X
the **antioxidants**
of **yellow peaches**

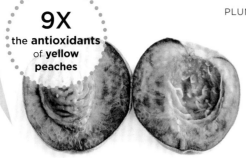

Antioxidants 5,801mg/g

Red

The romantically named 'blood peaches' are a collection of varieties whose flesh is naturally dyed deep red with anthocyanins, giving them up to an incredible nine times the antioxidant activity of the regular yellow forms, according to *The Journal of Agricultural and Food Chemistry*. In theory, you'd have to eat two pretty big punnets of yellow peaches to reap the antioxidant benefits of just one red one so trying something new could really pay off.

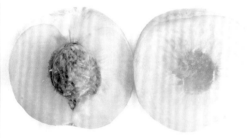

Antioxidants 1,048mg/g

White & yellow

The fascinating, and sometimes frustrating, thing about science is that every so often a finding comes along that breaks the general rules. For, despite having up to ten times more carotenoids than their white-fleshed cousins, yellow-fleshed peaches and nectarines don't actually have more overall antioxidants. This is because white-fleshed ones make up for their lack of carotenes with much higher levels of a polyphenol called chlorogenic acid, a powerful antioxidant that studies suggest may help blood pressure and even slow the absorption of sugars into the bloodstream. In fact, some studies even suggest white-fleshed types may have a nutritional edge, including a third more vitamin C on top of their 65 per cent higher antioxidant levels.

LOWEST ANTIOXIDANTS

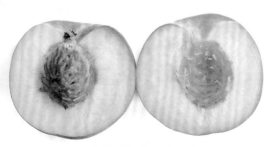

Antioxidants 637mg/g

PEACHES VS NECTARINES

What's the difference between a peach and a nectarine? Well, botanically, very little. They are both simply different cultivars of the same species, which essentially only vary in the genes that code for the fuzz on their skin. Beyond the fluff factor, studies show they are pretty much identical from a nutritional point of view. What can make a difference, as always, is their colour.

DITCH THE CANNED

OK, I'll admit it: I love canned peaches. And none of that 'in natural juice' stuff either – for full childhood-flashback foodie nostalgia, only heavy syrup will do. Too bad, then, that the act of peeling peaches for canning knocks their polyphenol content by 25 per cent. Another 30 per cent then leaches out of the fruit and into the canning liquid. Keep them on the shelf for 6 months (about the amount of time they can take to get to you) and they lose another 20 per cent. All in all, this slow chipping away at their phytonutrient content means that canned peaches can retain as little as half their original polyphenols and carotenes. Don't get me wrong, I still love scoffing them straight from the tin on hot summer days – I just don't kid myself they are as nutritious as the real deal.

GRAB THEM RIPE

My mate Rob hates peaches. It's a texture thing. He says he just can't stand their 'woolly, mealy' consistency. If you are like Rob, I implore you to try one thing: sidestep the 'ripen at home' packs and fork out just a little more on the 'ripe and ready to eat' kind. You see, when subjected to the chilly temperatures of commercial storage, unripe peaches undergo complex chemical reactions that can cause their internal tissues to break down – creating that familiar grainy-not-silky mouthfeel. If you've ever bought peaches that tend to go from rock-hard to mouldy, without ever actually ripening, it is likely that this 'chilling injury' is the cause.

Yet the exact same variety of peach harvested a little bit riper has much less risk of this happening, for reasons scientists are just beginning to understand. This increase in quality is, however, matched by a shorter shelf life and therefore higher price. I promise you, the improved texture and flavour are worth it, and frankly it is certainly cheaper than chucking whole trays of 'woolly' ones in the bin.

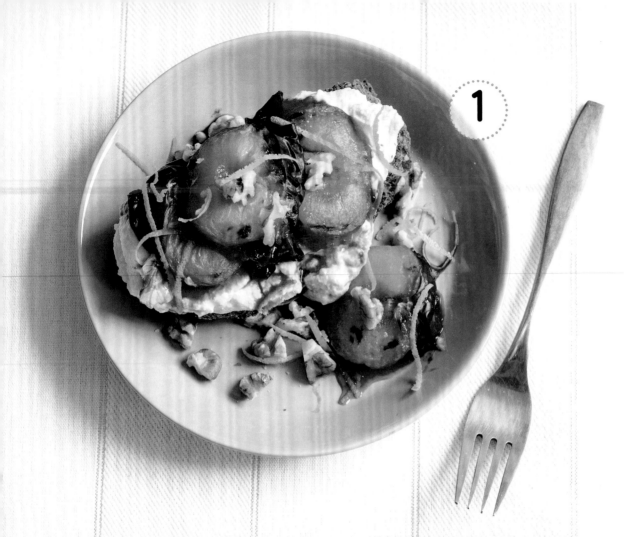

ROAST PLUMS WITH CINNAMON & CHILLI

Fifteen minutes in the oven has a magical effect on plums, concentrating flavours, caramelizing sugars and liberating healthy anthocyanin pigments trapped in their skins. Add a touch of spice and you have sticky, sweet goodness to boost the flavour and nutrition of everything from chicken salad to autumnal puddings. Yum.

SERVES 4
PREP TIME 10 MINUTES
COOK TIME 15 MINUTES

8 RIPE PLUMS, HALVED AND STONED
1 TBSP CLEAR HONEY
2 TBSP OLIVE OIL
1 TSP DICED CHILLI
½ TSP CINNAMON

PREHEAT the oven to 200°C/Gas Mark 6 and line a baking sheet with nonstick baking paper.

ARRANGE the plums, cut side up, on the prepared baking sheet, drizzle over the honey and oil and sprinkle with the chilli and cinnamon. Bake for 15 minutes.

HOW TO SERVE

(1) RICOTTA TOAST

Spread 200g **ricotta cheese** over 4 slices of warm **wholegrain sourdough toast**, then spoon over the **Roast Plums with Cinnamon & Chilli** and scatter with 50g chopped **walnuts** and finely grated **orange** zest.

(2) ROAST CHICKEN SALAD

Put 100g **watercress** in a serving bowl and add a handful of **pomegranate seeds**, ½ sliced **cucumber**, 2 sliced **spring onions** and a handful of **pecan nuts**. Arrange the **Roast Plums with Cinnamon & Chilli** over the salad and drizzle with 2 tbsp **olive oil** and 1 tbsp **balsamic vinegar**. Toss together, then top with 250g sliced **roast chicken**.

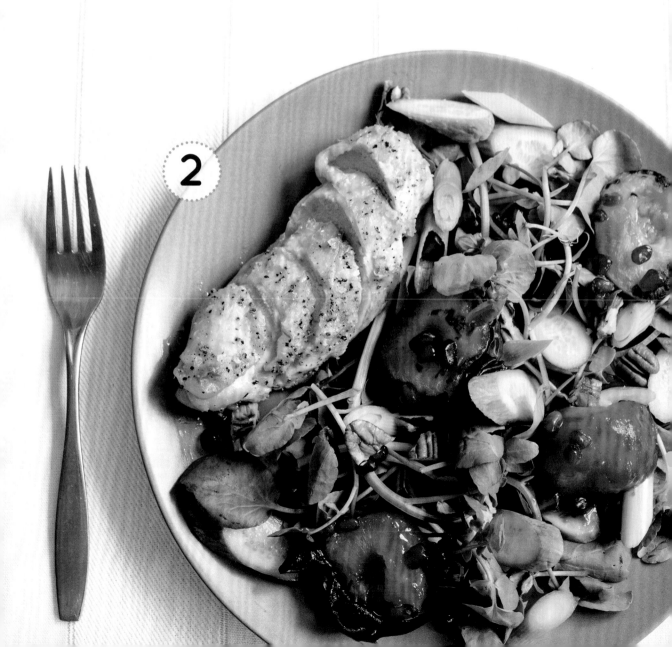

GRILLED PEACH, BEETROOT & FETA SALAD

Peaches don't just have to be the stuff of smoothies and fruit salads, their aromatic flavour and smooth texture work incredibly well in savoury dishes, too. Paired with tangy goats' cheese, salty Jamón Ibérico and peppery leaves, the sweetness of peaches makes this a salad that hits your taste buds from all sides.

SERVES 4

PREP TIME 20 MINUTES

COOK TIME 45 MINUTES

....

50G WALNUTS

4 COOKED BEETROOTS, CUT INTO WEDGES

4 PEACHES, HALVED, STONED AND CUT INTO WEDGES

50G FETA CHEESE, CRUMBLED

1 RED ONION, VERY FINELY SLICED

50G ROCKET LEAVES

50G WATERCRESS

80G JAMÓN IBÉRICO

1 QUANTITY ROAST CHICKPEA CROUTONS (SEE PAGE 198)

SALT AND PEPPER

CASHEW RANCH DRESSING

100G SPRING ONIONS, ROUGHLY CHOPPED

50G HONEY-ROASTED CASHEW NUTS

1 TBSP GRATED PARMESAN CHEESE

FINELY GRATED ZEST AND JUICE OF 1 LEMON

2 TBSP GARLIC MAYONNAISE

½ TSP ENGLISH MUSTARD

½ TSP WORCESTERSHIRE SAUCE

1 TBSP ROUGHLY CHOPPED DILL

1 TBSP ROUGHLY CHOPPED PARSLEY

½ TSP SALT

HEAT a nonstick frying pan over a medium-low heat and toast the walnuts for about 5 minutes, stirring frequently, until golden brown. Remove from the pan and set aside.

PREPARE the cashew ranch dressing. Blitz all the ingredients together in a food processor until smooth.

ARRANGE the all the salad ingredients on a serving plate and season with salt and pepper. Drizzle one-third of the dressing over the salad (the remainder can be stored in the fridge for up to 3 days) and serve.

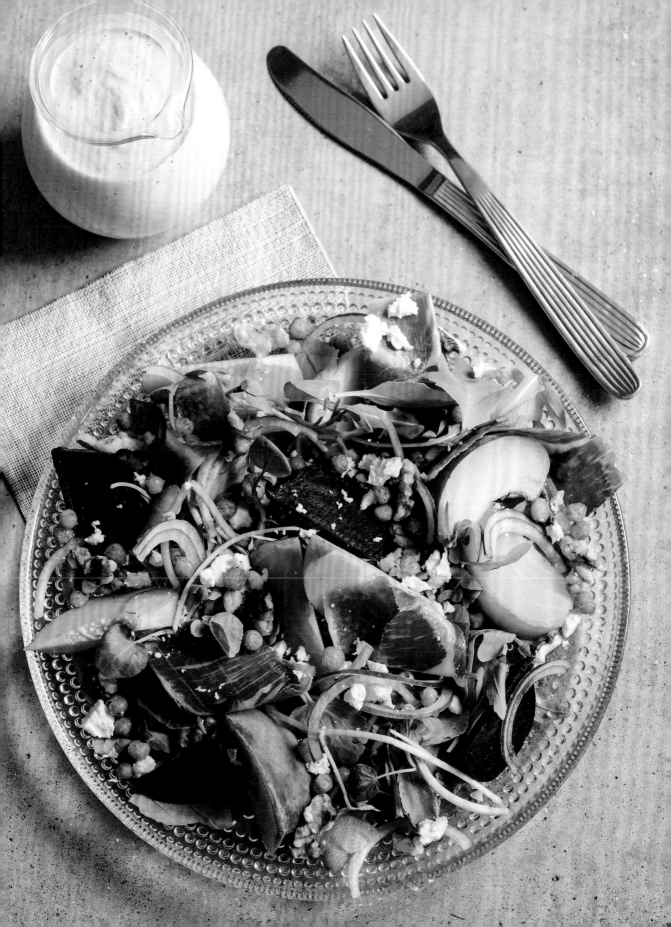

KIWIFRUIT

Twice the vitamin C content of an orange, as much fibre as a bowl of porridge and loaded with antioxidants like lutein and zeaxanthin, kiwifruit are bite-for-bite one of the most nutritionally dense fruit in the world. But the benefits don't end there.

♡ RESTFUL SLEEP

Kiwis are rich in a hormone called serotonin, which our brains produce to aid restful sleep and regulate mood, making them frequently cited in the press as 'great for insomniacs'. Indeed, one study published in the *Asia Pacific Journal of Nutrition* found that consuming 2 kiwifruit an hour before bed could significantly improve sleep onset, duration and quality in insomnia sufferers. The patients dozed off a third quicker, slept for 13 per cent longer and woke up in the night 30 per cent less. That's the equivalent of getting an hour's extra kip a night! And better-quality kip at that. OK, it was just one trial, but it's an intriguing start.

The weird thing is, however, the serotonin we ingest through food shouldn't be able to cross the blood–brain barrier to actually have an impact on our brain chemistry. Even if it did, pineapples contain nearly three times more serotonin and don't seem to have this effect. So the mechanism of how kiwis *may* work in this respect is still unknown. More research is needed to see if these results can be replicated and, if so, what it is in kiwis that might be causing this effect. In the meantime, insomniacs, there are worst after-dinner treats out there than a couple of kiwis.

♡ COMBATTING COLDS

Various compounds, from vitamin C and fibre to carotenes and polyphenols, have been shown to be beneficial to immune function. All of these also just so happen to be found neatly bundled up – in some pretty high doses – in the form of kiwifruit. So could eating kiwis boost immune function? Scientists have so far tested this theory in lab and animal studies with promising results, but human trials have been few and far between – until now! In one study from New Zealand's Massey University, preschool children (a high-risk group for catching coughs and colds) who ate 2 gold kiwis a day caught half the number of such illnesses. When it came to older people (another high-risk group) researchers found that regular gold kiwi consumption may not reduce the incidence of respiratory infections, but slashed the duration and severity of symptoms such as head congestion and sore throat.

♡ BLOOD PRESSURE QUELLING

Kiwifruit are a great source of potassium, an essential mineral that fewer than 2 per cent of people consume enough of. This is a huge shame as research suggests it may counteract the blood-pressure-raising effect of a high-salt diet. Research at the University of Oslo found that adding 3 kiwifruit to the daily diet of male smokers with hypertension could reduce their blood pressure significantly within 8 weeks, potentially reducing their risk of a cardiovascular event by approximately 10 per cent. Not quite as dramatic results as seen in foods like beetroot (see page 83), but not bad!

♡ DIGESTIVE HEALTH

Eating 2 green kiwis a day not only could keep you regular, but it also has been shown to significantly improve the digestion of patients with IBS, according to scientists at Taipei Medical University in Taiwan. With 2 kiwis containing as much fibre as a serving of a high-bran breakfast cereal, that isn't surprising!

KIWIS BITE BACK

Ever noticed an unpleasant tingling sensation on your lips and tongue after eating kiwis? That's caused by crystals of a compound called calcium oxalate that is naturally found in green kiwis. Their sharp edges irritate the lining of mucous membranes and can cause serious discomfort in people who are sensitive to them. Green kiwis contain 40 per cent more than gold forms and a whopping four times more than baby kiwifruit. If you are sensitive to this chemical, picking one of the other varieties could help, as can leaving them on the work surface for a few days to make sure they are fully ripe, as levels of calcium oxalate can halve during storage.

HIGHEST POLYPHENOLS AND SWEETER FLAVOUR

LOWEST POLYPHENOLS AND SOUREST FLAVOUR

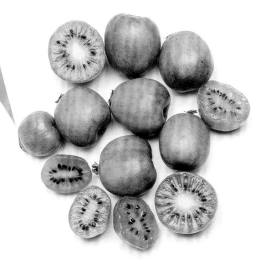

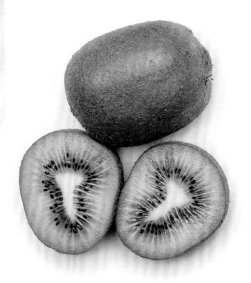

Baby kiwis (*Actinidia arguta*)

Über-cute mini kiwis the size of a grape with skin as smooth and thin as a cherry, these guys make up for their small stature by being true nutritional heavyweights. For starters, they have three times the vitamin C and betacarotene of the regular green type. They also contain twice the lutein, a carotene that is believed to protect the eye from age-related decline (see page 94), making it the richest dietary source of this nutrient among commonly consumed fruit. To top it all off, they are also much sweeter and richer in aromatic compounds than regular kiwis, making them taste almost like kiwi-flavour pick-and-mix sweets – more kiwi than kiwi. The only flaw these little beauties have is that their soft, berry-like texture means they have a much shorter shelf life. You won't find them on the shelves all year round, but boy are they worth it when you do.

Gold kiwis (*Actinidia chinensis*)

Gram for gram, the flesh of the gold kiwifruit has been found to contain significantly higher levels of polyphenols, plus 40 per cent more carotenes and 60 per cent more vitamin C than its green cousin. It even tastes sweeter, with a rich tropical fruit flavour all of its own. But to me, the real nutritional secret weapon of the gold kiwi is its fuzz-free skin. Without the irritating fibres on its surface, it can be eaten without peeling and this could be a game-changer as the skin contains three times the antioxidant activity of the flesh.

One study found that by doing this you would get 60 per cent more antioxidants per serving. As traditional like-for-like comparisons of these two kiwi varieties have not taken into account the edible skin of the gold variety, it is likely many under-report the potential nutritional value per serving of these golden wonders. In one clinical trial, volunteers who consumed either one or two gold kiwis a day for a month were found to have not only lower levels of triglycerides and higher resistance towards DNA damage, but also a reduced risk of forming blood clots.

Green kiwis (*Actinidia deliciosa*)

The vast majority of the world's kiwifruit sales are dominated by a single green variety called Hayward. Although it might be from a species called '*deliciosa*', compared to the other varieties it is really anything but. Not only does it contain far fewer nutrients and sugar, it also contains the highest amounts of unpleasant calcium oxalate.

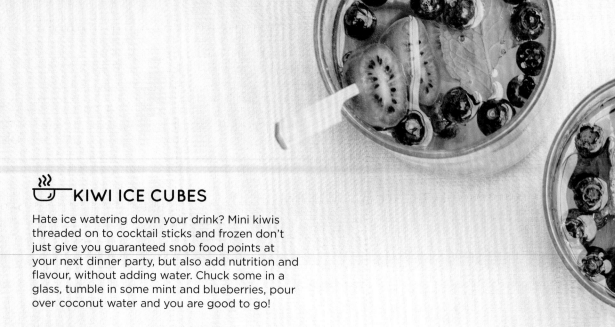

🍵 KIWI ICE CUBES

Hate ice watering down your drink? Mini kiwis threaded on to cocktail sticks and frozen don't just give you guaranteed snob food points at your next dinner party, but also add nutrition and flavour, without adding water. Chuck some in a glass, tumble in some mint and blueberries, pour over coconut water and you are good to go!

🍵 SALAD SAVIOUR

Winter salads can be boring, but kiwis can help with this, too. I find their sweet-tart flavour works great in savoury salads, with bitter leaves like radicchio, creamy mozzarella, salty persimmon and fresh blood oranges.

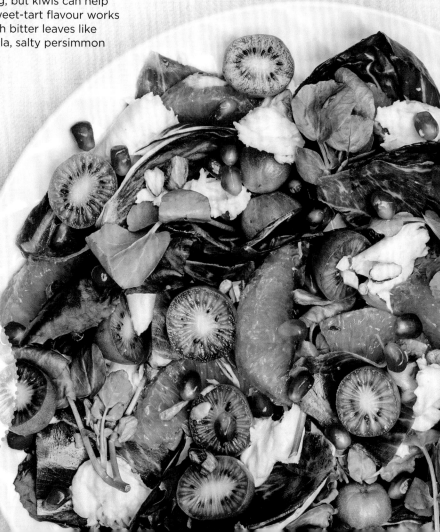

Baby kiwis have **3x** the **vitamin C** and **betacarotene, yet taste sweeter**

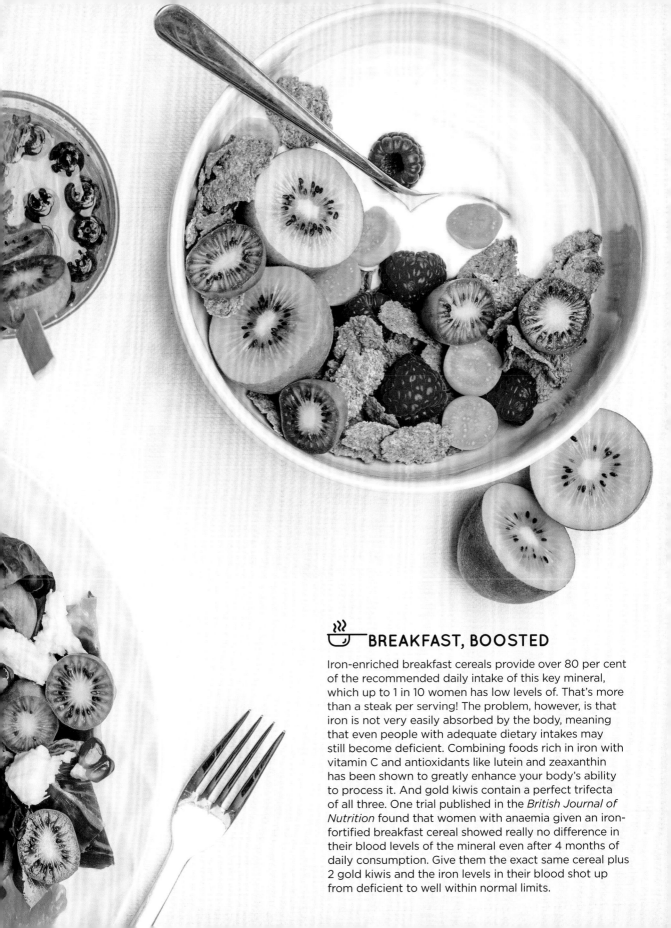

☕ BREAKFAST, BOOSTED

Iron-enriched breakfast cereals provide over 80 per cent of the recommended daily intake of this key mineral, which up to 1 in 10 women has low levels of. That's more than a steak per serving! The problem, however, is that iron is not very easily absorbed by the body, meaning that even people with adequate dietary intakes may still become deficient. Combining foods rich in iron with vitamin C and antioxidants like lutein and zeaxanthin has been shown to greatly enhance your body's ability to process it. And gold kiwis contain a perfect trifecta of all three. One trial published in the *British Journal of Nutrition* found that women with anaemia given an iron-fortified breakfast cereal showed really no difference in their blood levels of the mineral even after 4 months of daily consumption. Give them the exact same cereal plus 2 gold kiwis and the iron levels in their blood shot up from deficient to well within normal limits.

PASTA

Amid trendy carb-o-phobia, pasta has often been vilified as a sort of diabetic rocket fuel guaranteed to send blood sugar levels soaring out of control. Even worse, it contains (gasp!) gluten, which has put it right at the top of the wellness bloggers' ever-growing list of 'bad' foods. As always, however, the science tells a rather different story to the headlines. Pasta is actually one of the lowest glycaemic index values (see page 46) of all grain products, with a unique structure that makes the carbs it contains far more steadily released into the bloodstream. Take the same ingredients in identical quantities and bake them into bread, for example, and they trigger nearly double the spike in blood sugar, according to Sweden's Lund University.

🧺 BROWN IS BEST

Wholegrain pasta is far and away the most nutritious of all forms. Simply picking this over the regular kind will give you two and a half times the fibre and roughly twice the levels of pretty much every vitamin and mineral, including iron, thiamin and B vitamins. All this for 20 per cent fewer calories, too. According to the University of Sydney, it ranks higher on the 'satiety index', keeping hunger at bay for 60 per cent longer. It's a no-brainer, really.

What about the green and orange types? These are regular refined pastas coloured using a tiny amount of spinach or dried tomato powder, typically about 2–3 per cent. These look beautiful but are nutritionally very similar to plain white pasta.

🧺 PICK THICK & CHUNKY

Swedish researchers have found that the thickness to which pasta dough is rolled can have a noticeable impact on its GI. While the chunkiest linguine ribbons are in the medium range at 68 (similar to wholegrain bread), rolling the same dough to a thinner setting could drive its GI to a sky-high 87 (higher than sliced white). Similar findings were found by New Zealand researchers, who reported that the increasing number of passes through ever-tighter rollers freed up starch grains in pasta, making them easier to digest. While the researchers were quick to point out that these differences were relatively modest (say, in comparison to making bread out of the same ingredients), they could be 'somewhat more advantageous' to people managing diabetes, for example. And why not?

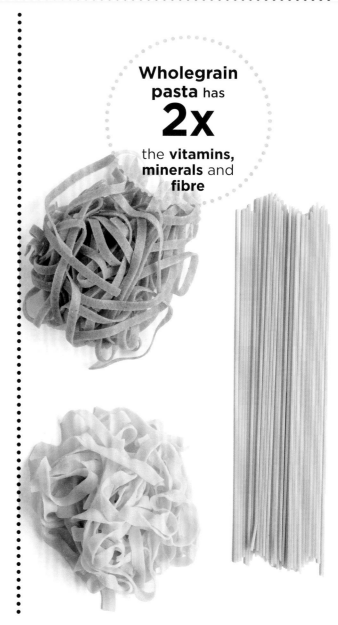

Wholegrain pasta has **2x** the **vitamins, minerals** and **fibre**

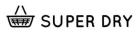 ## SUPER DRY

Dried pasta is not only much cheaper than the fancy fresh kinds, it also lasts pretty much indefinitely. And as the high temperatures it is subjected to in commercial drying trigger the protein molecules in the pasta to cross-link, creating a more rigid encapsulation of the starch grains, it seems the cheapest and longest lasting is also potentially a marginally healthier option.

BEANY BENEFITS

OK, so here is a bit of a curveball. Picking pasta not made from wheat at all, but low-calorie, nutrient-dense veg is probably the best option of all. No, no, wait. I don't mean those spiralized courgette abominations (frankly who on earth can call this 'pasta' with a straight face, I don't know), but those made from bean flour. There is a long tradition of this in East Asia, with a massive range of them exploding onto Western markets in the last few years. This pasta, surprisingly, has a taste and texture extremely similar to fancy egg pasta, with the extra protein in beans giving it that delicious firmer bite and a more elastic consistency. It cooks just as quickly as regular pasta, but doesn't tend to go soft and squishy if you forget it on the hob, either. No risk of a stodge-fest here.

Now we have got flavour and convenience out of the way, let's look at the nutritional stats. Being made from 100 per cent pure beans, bean-flour pasta contains over three times the protein, six times the fibre and 60 per cent fewer carbs per serving compared to wheat pasta. I am the first person to call out a health-food gimmick when I see one, but for me personally, they are a bit of a game-changer.

THE SECRET'S IN THE STRUCTURE

When the pasta is extruded under pressure into its various shapes, the proteins it contains form a microscopic matrix that traps the grains of starch between them, making it much harder for the digestive enzymes produced by our bodies to get at it. Compared to the fluffy sponginess of leavened bread, this dense lattice breaks down much more slowly, giving you a sustained release of energy with a GI value on a par with some fruit and vegetables. It isn't surprising really that this way of eating grain is a central part of the traditional Mediterranean diet, which research suggests may be one of the healthiest on earth. Pass the spaghetti!

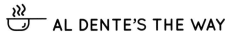 ## AL DENTE'S THE WAY

The funny thing about starch is that it essentially contains little or no calories until you cook it. As the key way by which plants store energy to help tide them over lean periods, plants use starch as a botanical battery precisely because it's a great method of locking up calories in a way that resists them being released. Applying water and heat through cooking is an ingenious human invention that changes the structure of these carbs into a gelatinized form that is much easier for our bodies to access. In many ways, cooking is a sort of technological pre-digestion, allowing us to get more from less. This means that cooking pasta al dente, with a very slight raw bite at its very core, will result in the same food having a lower GI by significantly reducing its digestibility compared to soft-cooked pasta. Indeed, this is exactly what public health bodies like the University of Sydney's Glycemic Index Foundation and the American Diabetes Association recommend.

COOK & CHILL

As with all starchy foods, cooking and then chilling pasta initiates a chemical reaction that converts part of its carbs into 'resistant starch' (see page 106). As this is essentially indigestible, not only are the total calories in the dish reduced, but also our bodies now treat this starch more like fibre, further lowering the effect of the dish on GI. This makes pasta salad potentially a lower GI choice to freshly cooked. I don't know about you, however, but there is only so much cold pasta I am willing to eat. To make this a more practical, everyday habit, it's got to work reheated.

By a wonderful stroke of coincidence, it turns out that the act of reheating cooked and cooled pasta not only retains these benefits, but can in fact lower its GI even further, reducing the rise in blood sugar by 50 per cent, according to one small pilot trial run by the University of Surrey. While more research is under way to establish if these findings are repeatable, they do reflect similar discoveries made in starchy veg like potatoes and sweet potatoes (see pages 49 and 53). Leftovers that are potentially healthier than the original dish? Why not!

NO-COOK PASTA SAUCES

If you're going to the effort of cooking your pasta the night before and reheating it, you might as well save yourself some time with a superfast no-cook sauce. Bung your chilled pasta in the microwave or blanch in hot water to warm through, toss one of the sauces below through it and you are good to go. Each of these sauces serves 1 person.

1 WATERCRESS & LEMON PESTO

Put a handful of chopped **watercress** and 2 tbsp **honey-roasted cashews** into a bowl, then stir in finely grated zest of ½ **lemon**, ½ **garlic clove** (chopped), 2 tbsp grated **Parmesan cheese** and 1 tbsp **olive oil**.

2 PUTTANESCA

Flake 150g **smoked trout** into a bowl, then add 2 tbsp sliced **black olives**, 1 tbsp **capers** and 10 halved **cherry tomatoes**. Top with finely grated zest of ½ **lemon**, 1 tsp chopped **chilli**, ½ **garlic clove** (chopped), 2 tbsp grated **Parmesan cheese** and 1 tbsp **olive oil**.

3 FRUIT & NUT

Defrost a handful of **frozen peas**, add to a bowl and mix together with 50g crumbled **Roquefort**, 50g toasted **flaked almonds** and 20g **sultanas**. Top with finely grated zest of ½ **orange**, 1 tsp chopped **dill** and 1 tbsp **olive oil**.

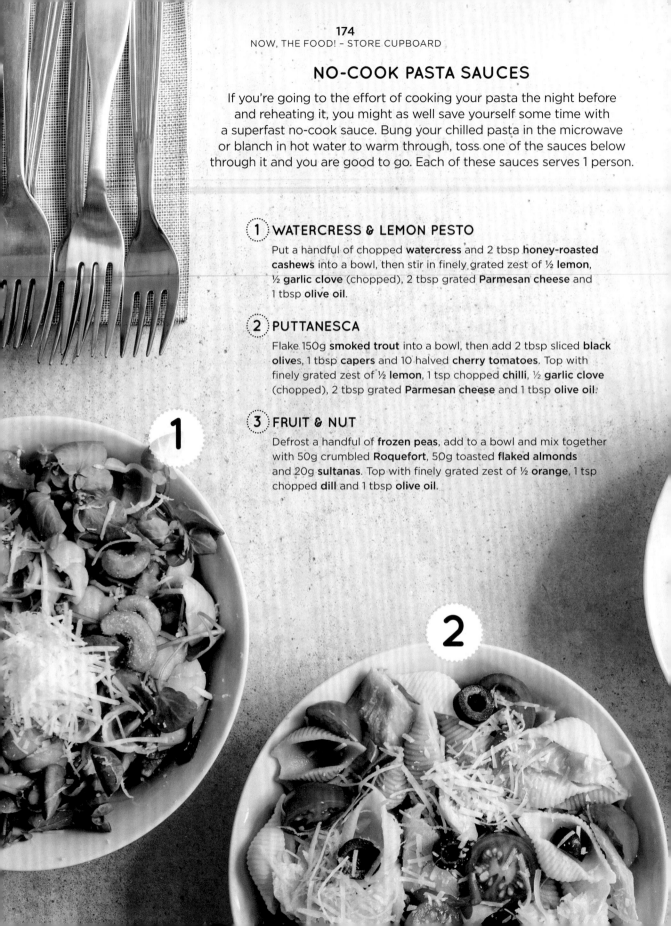

④ PRIMAVERA

Grate 1 **courgette** and finely slice 100g **asparagus** and tip into a bowl, then crumble in 50g **feta cheese**. Toss together with 1 tbsp **olive oil**, ½ **garlic clove** (minced), finely grated zest of ½ **lemon**, a handful of fresh **mint** and ½ tsp grated **nutmeg**.

⑤ TOMATO, WALNUT & ROCKET

Halve 10 **cherry tomatoes**, then tip into a bowl with 100g **roasted red peppers** (sliced) and a handful of **rocket**. Toss together with a handful of **fresh basil**, 2 tbsp grated **Parmesan cheese**, 1 tbsp chopped **walnuts** and 1 tbsp **olive oil**.

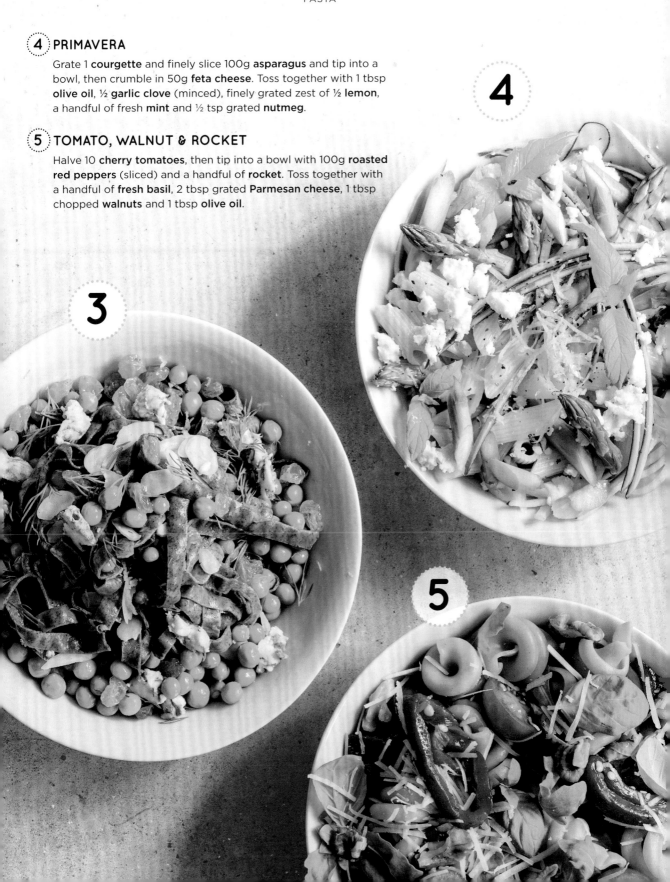

RICE

It might be the most widely eaten grain on earth, fuelling the bodies of billions, but by far the most popular variety – regular white rice – also happens to be one of the least nutritious. Yet armed with a little knowledge about which are the best varieties to pick *and* simple tricks on how to cook them, anyone can double rice's levels of a whole bunch of vitamins and minerals, halve its spike in blood sugar, send its fibre content soaring sixfold – and even slash its calories.

CONVERT TO CONVERTED

As with all carbs from spuds to pasta, chilling cooked rice for 12 hours results in a sizeable chunk of its carbs being converted to a substance called 'resistant starch' (see page 106), which can reduce its absorbable calories around 10 per cent and slow its impact on blood sugar.

There is, however, an even simpler way to take advantage of this same chemical reaction. Just picking parboiled rice at the supermarket may offer similar benefits. Also known as 'converted rice', this industrial process steams the grains under pressure while still in their husks, before being dried and packaged. Manufacturers do this as it gives the rice a longer shelf life and makes the grains more resistant to milling, but by coincidence it also has the effect of raising levels of resistant starch, knocking its GI by as much as 30 per cent, according to Danish research published in the *European Journal of Clinical Nutrition*. Harvard University makes an even bolder claim, reporting parboiled white rice to have the ridiculously low GI value of 38, almost half the values they report for regular white rice (GI 73) and putting it on a par with fruit and veg like carrots and apples. But the good news doesn't stop there. This pressure steaming also drives water-soluble nutrients like thiamine, niacin and riboflavin, as well as B vitamins, from the husk into the grain, boosting its nutrient levels. Parboiled rice is available for both brown and white forms and is well worth seeking out for the nutritional payback. Don't confuse it with 'easy cook rice', however, which is produced by a different process that has not shown the same benefits.

BROWN RICE, MADE BETTER

Before the advent of mechanical polishing, many people in Asia would traditionally soak brown rice in warm water for a day or so to soften the grain's chewier texture and give it a slightly sweet taste. This works by setting off the complex chemical reactions in rice seeds that happen when they sprout, creating a result that many people find tastier than plain old brown. Intriguingly, some research has also suggested that this same process can also significantly up its levels of fibre and essential minerals like zinc, potassium and magnesium. Test-tube and animal studies have also pointed at the idea that it may have anti-diabetic properties.

Although the jury might still be out on the wealth of fantastical health claims that are often ascribed to it, the improved texture and flavour might just be worth it if they persuade you into making the switch from white to brown. Sold as 'germinated' or 'sprouted' brown rice, this traditional Asian rice is now increasingly widely available in the West in health-food stores and fancier supermarkets, admittedly for quite a hefty price premium. The good news is, however, if you have an airing cupboard at home (and a bit of patience) it is extremely easy to make yourself. Simply pour the amount of rice you want to cook into a large mixing bowl and fill with enough water to just cover it. Put a plate or lid on top and sit it in a warm airing cupboard (or any location above 25°C) for a day or two. Then simply drain, rinse and cook as you would regular rice.

Twice
the impact on blood sugar

QUICKLY DIGESTED

SHORT-GRAIN WHITE RICE
GI value 90

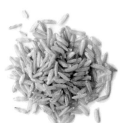

LONG-GRAIN WHITE RICE
GI value 72

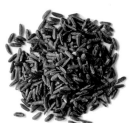

BROWN RICE
GI value 62

RED RICE
GI value 56

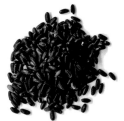

BLACK RICE
GI value 42

SLOWLY DIGESTED

Short-grain rice

The carbs in soft, squishy short-grain rice varieties come in the form of a super-easy-to-digest, gel-like starch called amylopectin, which offloads its sugars into the bloodstream almost as fast as straight-up table sugar. The very highest GI type of all appears to be the 'sticky' rice popular in Southeast Asian cooking, sometimes called 'glutinous rice' – with grains that are nearly 100 per cent pure amylopectin according to the supergeeks at the International Rice Research Institute.

In distant second place, and much lower than the 'sticky' types, come the traditional short-grain rice varieties used to make risotto, sushi, paella and rice pudding. These grains contain the same gel-like amylopectin as the sticky types, just mixed with a fluffier, harder-to-digest starch called amylose, which helps blunt their impact on blood sugar.

Pick a wholegrain form, however, and you knock its GI value even further, instantly turning this high GI food into a medium one. This is because the fibrous outer layer of the grain, which is polished off mechanically to make white rice, helps further slow digestion while simultaneously providing roughage to keep you feeling satisfied. In fact, each serving of brown rice contains a whopping six times more fibre than the same amount of white, according to the United States Department of Agriculture (USDA). Yet, funnily enough, as we'll see below, opting for wholegrain short-grain rice doesn't make anywhere near as much difference as just picking a long-grain variety.

Long-grain rice

The game-changer with long-grain rice is that it contains even more hard-to-digest amylose, giving it a slightly drier texture than the short-grain types, which also means the grains stay fluffy and separate when cooked. This includes varieties like regular white rice and jasmine rice. Some studies report that basmati rice, known for its particularly long, separated grains, is among the lowest GI of all this group, with an average GI bordering on the official definition of 'low'. The texture, it seems, is a dead giveaway.

As with short-grain rice, picking a brown variety will significantly lower the GI by adding a load of fibre. But the benefits of wholegrain don't stop there. Trapped in this fibrous layer also happens to be the bulk of the vitamins and minerals in rice, meaning wholegrain types can contain over two and a half times the antioxidants of white, according to Brazil's Federal University of Santa Maria. Going for brown will also give you twice the iron, vitamin B6 and magnesium of white, according to USDA.

Want to go one better? The same team of Brazilian geeks also found that fancy red rice comes packed with even more of the good stuff, boasting more than 11 times the polyphenol levels of white and the same GI as brown – a trend that research consistently pulls up in study after study.

Black rice

Lowest of the low in the GI stakes is rather conveniently the highest in terms of its antioxidant payload, packing more than about 14 times the polyphenols of the white stuff, according to the Brazilians, whose results reflect those of several previous studies. This is largely due to our old friends, the purple anthocyanin pigments found in fruit like blueberries. In fact, according to Louisiana State University, black rice may even rival blueberries in the antioxidant stakes, despite being much cheaper. Black rice even comes with a delicious nutty flavour. Make the swap for better flavour and better nutrition in every way.

BLACK RICE BOWL

Most recipes for black rice treat it in the same way as risotto rice (Italian style). But frankly, I can't be bothered with the slow stirring and gradual additions of ladlefuls of stock – especially when bunging it all in at once (Asian style) works just as well. You can serve this with any toppings you fancy, but here is a combo of my favourites.

SERVES 2

PREP TIME 10 MINUTES

COOK TIME ABOUT 45 MINUTES

. . . .

500ML VEGETABLE STOCK

200G BLACK RICE

1 RED ONION, FINELY DICED

1 GARLIC CLOVE, MINCED

1 TBSP EXTRA VIRGIN OLIVE OIL

TOPPINGS

2 READY-COOKED CHICKEN BREASTS,
SLICED

200G CHERRY TOMATOES, HALVED

50G PINEAPPLE ACHAR (SEE PAGE 160)

½ AVOCADO, PEELED AND SLICED

50G ROASTED CASHEW NUTS

SMALL HANDFUL OF ROCKET LEAVES

1 LIME, FINELY DICED
(PEEL AND ALL)

BRING the stock to the boil in a saucepan, add the rice and onion, then reduce the heat, cover and simmer for about 40–45 minutes until the rice is tender and all the liquid has been absorbed.

STIR in the garlic and olive oil and toss together, then spoon into 2 serving bowls.

ADD the toppings to each bowl and serve.

BLACK RICE PUDDING

One of my favourite breakfasts, this recipe is based on the most traditional Chinese way of eating black rice, which is a sort of rice pudding slightly slackened out with coconut milk. I have shamelessly Westernized it by adding fruit and yogurt to make it even healthier.

SERVES 2

PREP TIME 10 MINUTES

COOK TIME 50 MINUTES

. . . .

200G BLACK RICE

500ML WATER

100ML COCONUT MILK

1 TSP VANILLA EXTRACT

2 TBSP BROWN SUGAR

1 TSP MIXED SPICE

½ TSP SALT

TOPPINGS

CHOPPED FRUIT, SUCH AS MANGO
AND KIWIFRUIT

CHOPPED PISTACHIO NUTS

COCONUT MILK YOGURT (OPTIONAL)

COMBINE all the pudding ingredients in a saucepan and bring to the boil over a medium-high heat. Reduce the heat and simmer, uncovered, for 45 minutes, or until the rice is tender, stirring occasionally. Feel free to add extra water if needed, a splash at a time, especially towards the end of the cooking time.

SPOON into serving bowls and serve topped with chopped fruit and pistachios and a spoonful of coconut milk yogurt, if liked.

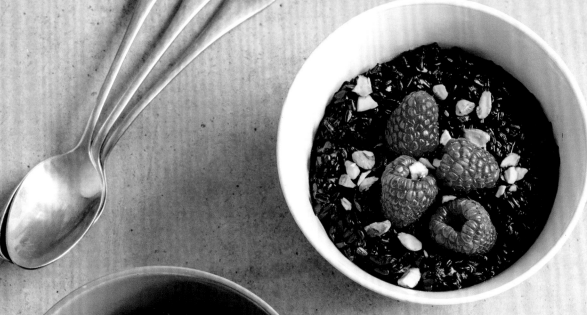

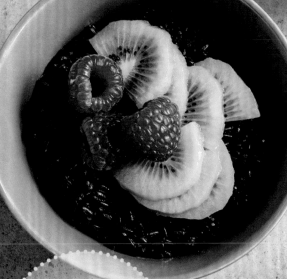

Get
14x
the heart-healthy
polyphenols
when you pick
black rice

Black rice
has the lowest
impact on blood
sugar of all rice

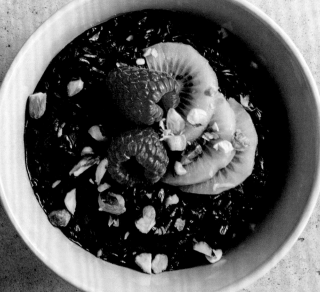

SAFFRON RICE & BEANS

My lovely auntie Monica makes the best rice and beans in the universe. It turns out this classic combo is as healthy as it is tasty, too, with a growing body of research demonstrating that pulses like peas, beans and lentils can blunt the impact of even super-high GI white rice on blood sugar by as much as 50 per cent when eaten together (see also page 193). These carb-quelling effects can last several hours, helping reduce the impact of carbs eaten at your next meal, even the next day!

The protein boost you get from 'cutting' rice with pulses helps keep you fuller for longer and that is before we even get on to all the extra polyphenols and flavour. As beans contain fewer calories and carbs, replacing part of your rice with them could even start to make an impact on your waistline over the long term. Talk about a win-win situation!

SERVES 4
PREP TIME 15 MINUTES
COOK TIME 45–50 MINUTES

1 TBSP OLIVE OIL

1 ONION, FINELY SLICED

2 CARROTS, GRATED

2 AUBERGINES, DICED

250G BROWN BASMATI RICE, RINSED

2 TSP SAFFRON THREADS

¼ TSP CINNAMON

500ML CHICKEN OR VEGETABLE STOCK

400G CAN BLACK BEANS, RINSED AND DRAINED

50G DRIED SOUR CHERRIES

100G SHELLED PISTACHIO NUTS

1 TBSP ROUGHLY CHOPPED PARSLEY

50G POMEGRANATE SEEDS

HEAT the oil in a large saucepan, add the onion, carrots and aubergine and fry gently for 10 minutes until golden.

STIR the rice, saffron and cinnamon into the vegetables and fry for 2–3 minutes. Add the stock, black beans and sour cherries and mix well, then slowly bring to the boil.

COVER with a lid and simmer for 25–30 minutes until the liquid is absorbed and the rice is tender.

SPRINKLE with the pistachios, parsley and pomegranate seeds and serve.

BEAN 'EM UP

Mixing a can of beans into cooked rice is hardly a massive inconvenience, *but* for truly lazy cooks out there (me included) there's an even simpler way to do this. Pair up slow-cooking brown rice and quick-cooking pulses like lentils and you can just bung the whole lot in the same pan and simmer it up in one go.

For two people, combine 100g brown rice with 100g black, green or brown lentils (sadly, red are too squishy to work) and 400ml water or stock in a saucepan. Whack it on the hob and once the whole lot reaches the boil, lower the heat, cover the pan and simmer for 25 minutes until tender. Hey presto! You've slashed the carbs and calories and pumped up the protein for no extra work. Thanks, Auntie Monica!

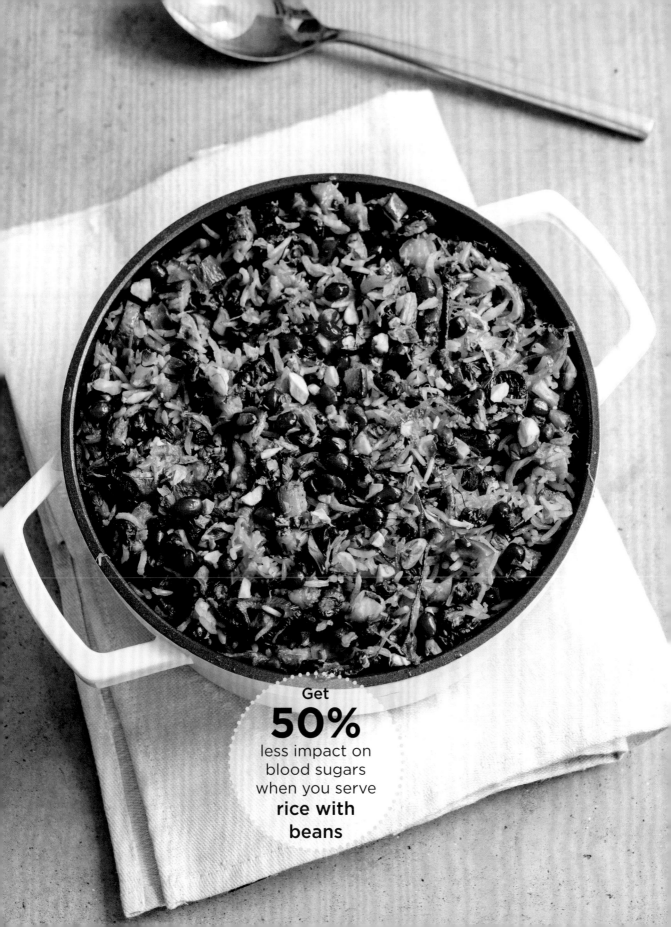

Get
50%
less impact on
blood sugars
when you serve
**rice with
beans**

OATS & BARLEY

Oats are in many ways the ultimate wholegrain. For starters, it is almost impossible to find them sold any other way, in stark contrast to rice, wheat and barley, which are much more commonly consumed in a heavily refined form. Oats are also higher in protein, calcium and essential fatty acids than most other grains. But what really sets them apart from all others – at least in terms of piquing the interest of food scientists – is their concentrated dose of a substance called beta-glucan. It has been proven by a stack of studies over decades that, with regular consumption, this soluble fibre reduces cholesterol. Out of all the potential health claims for individual foods, the evidence here is about as iron-clad as it gets.

♡ CHOLESTEROL BUSTING

After reviewing the findings of 37 scientific studies that found consuming just 3g of beta-glucan from oats each day could reduce cholesterol by between 5 and 10 per cent, in 1997 the US Food and Drug Administration passed a landmark piece of legislation. This allowed oat products to carry a health claim on their packaging stating their consumption could reduce cholesterol and therefore the risk of heart disease – the first-ever ruling of its kind.

A fall of this magnitude might seem small, but it is statistically associated with up to a 38 per cent reduction in the risk of heart disease at age 50. With high cholesterol affecting over a third of all Americans, this is a pressing concern. Since the 90s there have been at least two follow-up reviews that pooled together the findings of more recent studies. Both have simply served to reinforce the scientific consensus. Eating oats lowers cholesterol. Fact.

When beta-glucan hits your digestive tract it starts to absorb water, forming a thick, gel-like substance a bit like wallpaper paste. It's this mechanical property of beta-glucan that is believed to be behind its cholesterol-lowering properties. By trapping both the cholesterol in our food and that manufactured by our own bodies in its sticky quagmire, this fibrous gel prevents it from being absorbed into the bloodstream.

To hit the daily target of 3g of beta-glucan, you need to consume about 60g of rolled oats, an amount often described by public health authorities as between two and four portions a day. This sounds an awful lot. So I got the scales out, preparing to be daunted. It turns out 60g of rolled oats is barely enough to make an average cereal-bowlful of porridge, providing you with a modest 400 calories. Easily achievable. I hate to think how small the servings of public officials' breakfasts are!

♡ CONTROLLING BLOOD SUGAR, & EVEN BODY WEIGHT?

The very same property of beta-glucan believed to lower cholesterol is also thought to slow the absorption of sugar from our food, with some (but by no means all) studies reporting that oat consumption can prevent spikes in blood glucose, helping keep us feeling fuller for longer, and by extension even aiding weight management. Woohoo!

For example, in one small double-blind, randomized trial of overweight and obese men and women, researchers at Taiwan's Chung Shan Medical University found that almost 90 per cent of the subjects consuming an oat-based cereal every day for 12 weeks lost a significant amount of weight. But that's not all. Their findings echoed those of a previous trial in lab rats, right down to the reduction in their waistlines, a 20-point drop in cholesterol and even an improvement in liver function.

If this sounds almost too good to be true, how do the findings compare across the board? Well, in a 2014 review of trials investigating the impact of oat consumption in diabetics, a Brazilian team did indeed find that when viewed as a whole there was good evidence to suggest a significant reduction in blood sugar. Other similar reviews, such as one at University College Dublin, however, reported that the findings of the studies have so far been highly variable and contradictory. The jury may be out for now, and many more trials are needed before any firm conclusions can be made. In the meantime, however, I tuck into oats for breakfast every day and pray for a miracle.

🧺 WHOLE OATS

Pick three different packages off a supermarket shelf, all of which contain only 100 per cent wholegrain oats, and surprisingly their effect on satiety and blood sugar can be dramatically different. This is because how the grains are processed – in particular, how finely they are rolled, chopped up or otherwise broken down – can have an enormous impact on how your body processes them according to a review of more than 100 studies published in the *British Journal of Nutrition*.

This may explain why studies on the effect of eating oats on blood sugar are so variable. It's the *type* of oats that counts. Essentially, it appears the more intact the grain, the less our digestive enzymes are able to get at the starch within, resulting in a much slower rate of digestion – blunting their impact on blood sugar and, by extension, likely keeping you satiated for much longer. Here's how it breaks down:

Instant oats

In instant oats the individual oat grains are rolled flat to create flakes and then blitzed into a fine dust, almost the consistency of flour. These tiny fragments have a much greater surface area and a more porous texture, soaking up water in a fraction of the time, making them super-quick to cook. Unfortunately, the properties that make these so easy to prepare also make them super-easy to digest. Go for instant types and the carbs can hit your bloodstream as quickly as white bread or even plain old table sugar! As many of these also come with a hefty added dose of the sweet stuff to give them irresistible kid-appeal, what sounds like a healthy breakfast might not be so great after all. The quick-cook types, also known as porridge oats or thin flake oats, are essentially the same as the instant types, just broken up a little more coarsely. This results in slightly larger chunks that take a tad longer to cook and therefore digest, with a GI of 71. They are still super-high GI compared to other types, though.

Jumbo oats

Take the exact same rollers used to make quick-cook oats and set them a tiny bit further apart and something magical happens. The thicker, chunkier flakes that result tend to stay intact, dramatically lowering their effect on blood sugar, while giving them (to me at least) a much more satisfying bite. This small tweak turns what was once a high GI food into low GI one – without any change in ingredients. Weirdly, granolas and mueslis – despite their added sugars in the form of dried fruit, honey and in some cases table sugar – have a similar GI to jumbo oats according to the study (see 'Go for Muesli', page 184).

Pinhead oats

Sometimes known as steel-cut oats, these are whole oat grains that, instead of being squished flat, are roughly chopped by big steel blades on a rolling drum. Essential hipster fodder, they are becoming increasingly trendy in achingly cool cafés that pepper words like 'artisan' and 'heritage' through their menus. Despite all my eye rolling, I find they have a lovely nutty flavour and satisfying bite. But they take ages to cook, requiring overnight soaking and up to 25 minutes of simmering and constant stirring. After all that effort, they have a GI equivalent to that of jumbo oats, which cook two and a half times faster. Frankly, who has the time? Tasty, but I think I'll leave cooking them to the ironic beard brigade.

SLOWLY DIGESTED ➤ **QUICKLY DIGESTED**

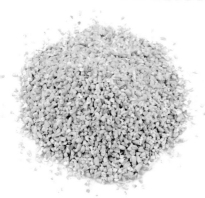

PINHEAD OATS
GI value 53

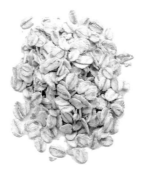

JUMBO OATS
GI value 55

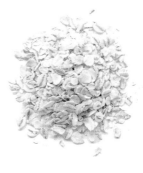

INSTANT OATS
GI value 75

OAT BRAN

This unpromising-looking powdery stuff is the most nutrient-dense outer layer of the grain that is removed when the oats are milled to make flour. It not only contains more B vitamins and iron than regular oats, but also packs a greater amount of healthful fibre – including 50 per cent more beta-glucan. Its small particle size makes it super-quick to cook, too, with its masses of soluble fibre giving it a deliciously smooth, creamy texture, despite it having a whopping 40 per cent fewer calories than regular oats. I was genuinely surprised at how tasty and convenient it is.

These benefits have been reflected in the results of at least one clinical trial. Published in the *Journal of the American Medical Association*, this reported that after 6 weeks of scoffing porridge made from either oats or oat bran, all participants showed a significant reduction in their cholesterol. But those in the bran group showed a 57 per cent edge over the oat eaters, a result that the researchers attributed to the higher levels of beta-glucan in the bran.

You can use oat bran as a direct replacement for rolled oats to make porridge, cooking it exactly as you would normally do. Alternatively, you can combine the two as a cheat's way to enrich regular oats, which still looks and tastes virtually identical. It also works well blitzed into smoothies and even simmered down in soups, to add a thicker, creamier texture with a boost of healthful fibre.

BARLEY'S BETTER

Barley, a close relative of oats, can contain as much as double the beta-glucan of its more celebrated cousin. It has a very similar flavour, too. So why aren't we all eating barley flakes instead of oats? Well, it's probably because most modern varieties tend to have so many of their outer layers polished off to remove their inedible hull, that their nutrient levels are knocked for six. This process, similar to that which creates white rice, results in the 'pearl barley' that dominates supermarket shelves. Sadly, all barley you have ever eaten is likely to have been a robbed of its wholegrain status.

That was, however, until the revived interest in ancient varieties of barley, which happen to produce no hull, started to bring these old 'hull-less' or 'naked' forms back to the market. Although they come with a range of trade names, the word 'wholegrain' on any of them is a sure giveaway. Rolled barley can be used in exactly the same way as oats, and comes packing a whole lot more of the good stuff. Wholegrain barley is also sold unrolled as fully intact grains (often called 'pot barley'), much like rice, and can be used in a very similar way.

In Italy wholegrain barley is sometimes used as a substitute for risotto rice to make 'orzotto' (*orzo*

meaning 'barley' in Italian). Making the swap does involve a little more waiting around, as wholegrain barley takes about 45 minutes to cook, versus a mere 20 minutes for rice, but you will be rewarded for your patience with over six times more fibre and twice the protein gram for gram. Unlike risotto rice, it doesn't require constant stirring either, making it great for lazy individuals like me! I'm happy to let it simmer in the background while I kick back on the sofa at the end of the day, in exchange for incredible flavour, a big nutritional boost and less work.

NUKE UP SOME NUTRITION

The type of oats you pick might have a huge impact on how they affect blood sugar levels, but this is only half the story. The way you choose to cook and serve them is what really seals the deal. When researchers at the Canadian government's Food Research Centre compared the nutritional impact of microwaving to conventional cooking on oats, they found a surprising difference in the amount of soluble starch in the end results – this is basically how much of the calorie-rich carbs are liberated from the grain by the cooking process and turned into a liquid form that is easily absorbed by the body. The fact that microwaving involved far less stirring, according to the researchers, meant that the grains were broken up less and the water wasn't quite as able to penetrate the grain, causing about 40 per cent less starch to be released. What does that mean for you? Well, as most of the calories in oats come from this starch, slashing the amount that is released is likely to significantly reduce the calories available in the finished dish. The insoluble starch that results now essentially acts like fibre, teaming up with the already sky-high fibre content of oats to make you feel fuller for longer, help keep you regular and even boost friendly gut bacteria.

GO FOR MUESLI

Want to go one better? Simply don't cook your oats at all. This reduces their calories and GI even further, while upping their fibre-like resistant starch (see page 106). This explains why muesli (which is eaten uncooked) had a similar GI rating to plain oats cooked up into porridge, despite containing a far larger dose of sugar from all the added dried fruit. The best bit? There are no more excuses for not having time to cook up a bowl of porridge in the morning because muesli is the ultimate instant food. Want a super-easy, low-cost recipe for a homemade version that tastes better than anything from the shops? I just happen to have a recipe on page 190.

PIMP YOUR PORRIDGE

Ever heard that old adage that a bowlful of porridge keeps you full right up until lunch? Is it me, or is that just a great big hoax? A steaming bowl of porridge might seem a comforting breakfast at 7am when I am dashing out the door, but just two hours later it has me ravenous and reaching for the nearest biscuit (a bit of an own goal there).

This isn't a surprise either. The 'average' 40g serving of oats simmered with 275ml semi-skimmed milk contains 271 calories: that's only about 10 per cent of the calories I need a day! Fortunately, there are things you can do about this. Bolt on some extras and you could have more nutritious, better-tasting porridge to keep mid-morning hunger at bay.

Protein

Serve your oats with a side of creamy Greek yogurt, either as porridge or with muesli, and you'll have significantly raised their filling protein content. Not a fan of the Greek stuff? A generous dollop of fromage frais with your oats will also seriously pump up the protein. Even cottage cheese (I know this sounds weird, but it totally works) can be delicious with a bowl of muesli instead of milk, alongside sliced fruit or a spoonful of jam to balance out its mild saltiness.

Fibre

Swap oats for oat bran or barley and you'll instantly up the filling fibre factor (including, of course, the heart-healthy beta-glucan). If you are a traditionalist at heart, simply 'cutting' the rolled oats with a sneaky scoop of either will help raise this, too, without you even noticing. Finally, adding a great big handful of fresh fruit, like berries, sliced apples, figs or, well, anything you like really, will send the phytonutrient levels soaring.

Healthy fats

Nuts and seeds contain not only protein, but also heart-healthy fats, boosting both flavour and nutrition. Fancy pecans and pistachios are my favourite muesli additions, but when it comes to porridge only a dollop of old-school chunky peanut butter will do. Pair this up with a slathering of my Blackberry & Cabernet Freezer Jam (see page 132) and you have a peanut butter and jam porridge worth getting out of bed for even on the darkest February day.

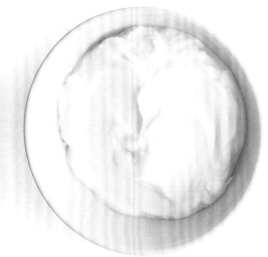
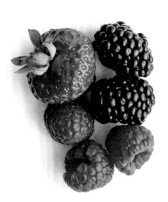
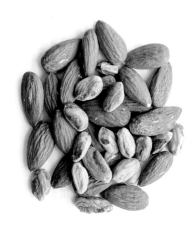

BARLEY RISOTTO BOWLS

Aside from its impressive health credentials, wholegrain barley is cheaper and less stodgy than risotto rice. It's also almost impossible to overcook and you can even bung the liquid in all at once, without hours of stirring. Pop everything in a pan, put your feet up for 45 minutes, give it a stir and it's done.

SERVES 4

PREP TIME 10 MINUTES

COOK TIME 1 HOUR

....

2 RED ONIONS, FINELY DICED

1 BAY LEAF

400G WHOLEGRAIN BARLEY (OFTEN SOLD AS 'POT BARLEY')

100ML WHITE WINE

1 LITRE CHICKEN OR VEGETABLE STOCK

200ML MILK

50G PARMESAN CHEESE, GRATED

2 TBSP OLIVE OIL

2 GARLIC CLOVES, MINCED

PUT the onions, bay leaf, barley, wine, stock and milk in a large saucepan – adding the milk last will stop it splitting when it hits the wine. Bring to the boil then cover, reduce the heat and simmer for 45 minutes, or until the barley is tender.

STIR through the Parmesan, oil and garlic, spoon into serving bowls and serve.

Barley has TWICE the protein and 6X more fibre than rice

HOW TO SERVE

1) GREEK WEEKEND BREAKFAST

Top each **Barley Risotto Bowl** with a boiled **egg** (halved), roast **cherry tomatoes**, sliced **cucumber**, pitted **black olives**, 1 **thyme** sprig, crumbled **feta cheese** and Pink Pickled Onions with Lime & Bay (see page 64).

2) SALMON & AVO WORKING LUNCH

Top each **Barley Risotto Bowl** with sliced **avocado**, chopped **dill**, **smoked salmon** strips, steamed **asparagus** and a slice of **lemon**.

3) WILD MUSHROOM SUPPER WITH FRIENDS

Stir 1 handful of **frozen peas**, 20 sliced and sautéed **shiitake mushrooms** and 2 tbsp **sherry** through the risotto 5 minutes before the end of the cooking time. Top each bowl with a drizzle of **truffle oil**, 1 tbsp **mascarpone** and a handful of **rocket** and season with **black pepper**.

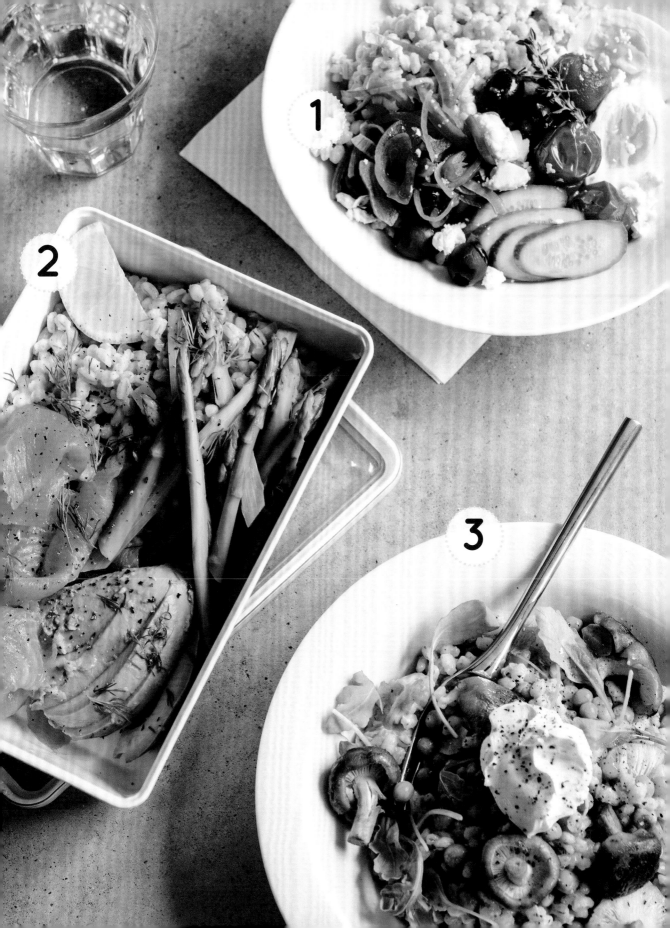

REFRIGERATOR OATS

No time to sit around stirring a pan of oats first thing each morning? Me neither! Then praise the foodie gods for refrigerator oats – mix everything together the night before, bung it in the fridge, soak overnight and it'll be there waiting for you to grab and go in the morning. Not cooking oats reduces the total number of calories you can absorb from them, while keeping you feeling fuller for longer. I like to top this with pecans, blueberries and goji berries, but you can use any fruit or nuts you like.

SERVES 1

PREP TIME 5 MINUTES, PLUS OVERNIGHT SOAKING

60G JUMBO ROLLED OATS

50ML MILK, PLUS EXTRA TO SERVE

100G GREEK YOGURT

1 RED APPLE, GRATED

¼ TSP MIXED SPICE

1 TSP CLEAR HONEY

2 TBSP SULTANAS

TOPPINGS

FRESH FRUIT

CHOPPED NUTS

MIX all the ingredients together in an airtight plastic container and leave to soak in the fridge overnight.

SERVE topped with the fruit and nuts.

VARIATIONS

1

MANGO & COCONUT

Make the **oat mixture** as above and stir through 30g **desiccated coconut**, then soak as above. Serve topped with 100g cubed **mango** and 1 large peeled and sliced **kiwifruit** and 1 tbsp **desiccated coconut**.

2

CARROT & WALNUT

Make the **oat mixture** as above and stir through 50g grated **carrot**, then soak as above. Serve topped with 2 tbsp extra **yogurt**, 20g grated **carrot** and 25g **walnuts**. This might sound weird, but it totally works.

3

APPLE & POMEGRANATE

Make the **oat mixture** as above and stir through 1 grated **apple**, then soak as above. Serve topped with 2 tbsp chopped **pistachio nuts** and 2 tbsp **pomegranate seeds**.

This recipe is so thick and substantial you can eat it with a fork. The breakfast of champions!

Each serving contains the full **3g** dose of heart-healthy **beta glucan** you need to lower cholesterol

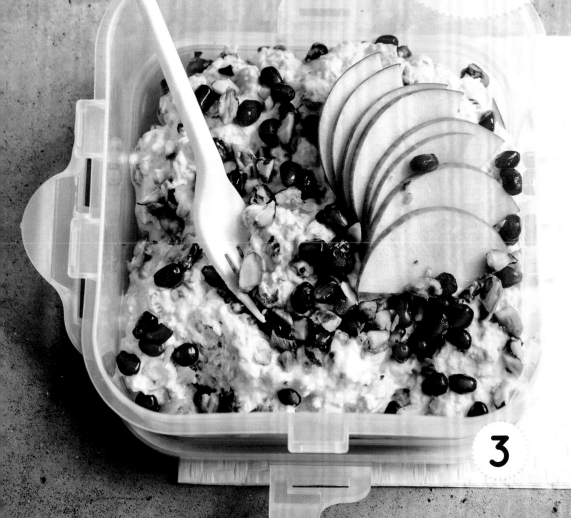

3

HOMEMADE BLUEBERRY & APPLE MUESLI

I love muesli, but getting hold of a good one can be expensive, which is such a shame as it is so easy to make your own cheapskate version. Being a pedantic geek, I actually crunched the numbers here, and found that on average this bootleg version cost me less than half the price of shop-bought and took me a grand total of 5 minutes to make enough for a week of breakfasts, with each serving containing more than my daily target 3g of beta-glucan.

Bored with having the same one every morning? Make up the same base and tweak the final ingredients to make a bunch of smaller batches in ziplock bags and you can have a different flavour every day. Here's a breakdown of my favourite formula, plus a couple of variations.

MAKES 7 SERVINGS
PREP TIME 5 MINUTES

BASIC BLUEBERRY MIX

500G ROLLED OATS, OR A 50:50 MIX OF ROLLED OATS AND ROLLED BARLEY

100G OAT BRAN

150G DRIED APPLES, CHOPPED

100G PITTED DATES, CHOPPED

50G FLAKED ALMONDS

100G DRIED BLUEBERRIES

1 HEAPED TBSP CINNAMON

FILL a large Kilner jar or airtight plastic container with the oats, barley, if using, and oat bran. Add the remaining ingredients and seal, then give it a good shake and you are good to go! Your mix will keep for up to 6 months stored in a cool, dry place.

This also makes **great porridge** in the winter months. Just whack it in the microwave for 3 minutes, stirring half way through.

SWEET CINNAMON
Some studies have suggested that cinnamon *might* also help control blood sugar. Combined with oats, you could get a theoretical double whammy – it's just as well they taste so good together.

VARIATIONS

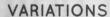 **APRICOT & GINGER**

Make the basic mix as opposite, replacing the dried blueberries with 100g **dried apricots** and 1 tsp **ground ginger**. Top each serving with 1 sliced **fresh apricot** and 25g sliced **stem ginger**.

② **STRAWBERRY & VANILLA**

Make the basic mix as opposite, replacing the dried blueberries with 100g **freeze-dried strawberries** and 1 tsp **vanilla powder.** Top each serving with 4–5 **fresh strawberries** and 25g chopped **pecan nuts**.

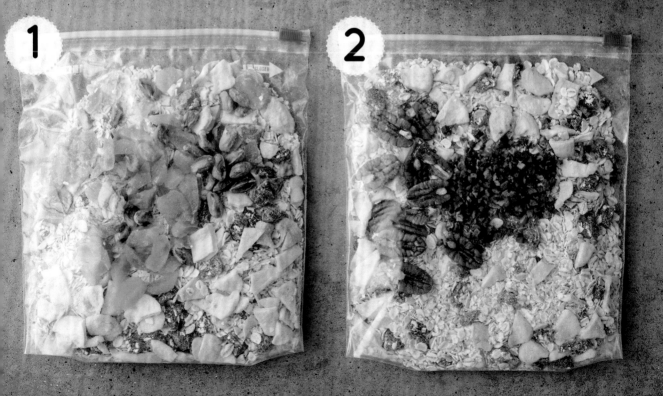

BEANS & PULSES

Rich in potassium, magnesium, iron and zinc, beans also come packed with loads of fibre and polyphenols, cramming an awful lot of nutrition into a super-low-calorie food. One of the few vegetables that is also an excellent protein source, they combine the best of both worlds in a cheap, convenient format. And yet in the Western world we consume precious few of them, with over 95 per cent of Americans (whose diet is becoming increasingly representative of many around the globe) not making the government recommended intake of just a modest 80g a day.

 ## OVERALL HEALTH

Why does that matter? Well, a study published in the *Asia Pacific Journal of Clinical Nutrition* by an international team of researchers may give some insight. It tracked the diets of hundreds of elderly people in Japan, Sweden, Greece and Australia and found that eating beans and pulses was linked to a 7–8 per cent reduction in the risk of death for every 20g increase in consumption. The higher the level of your bean consumption, the healthier you are likely to be, statistically speaking at least. But isn't this true of all fruit and veg? Well, in fact, the study found that tucking into beans was the single most important dietary predictor of survival in older people, regardless of where they lived, with all other food groups not found to be consistently significant.

 ## DIABETES & CHOLESTEROL

One widely demonstrated phenomenon that might lie behind these effects is the ability of beans to slow the absorption of sugars in high-carb meals, preventing spikes in blood glucose, potentially keeping you fuller for longer. Aside from their rich content of protein and fibre, which have a satiating effect, beans also contain chemicals that block the action of an enzyme called alpha-amylase, which is responsible for the digestion of starch. With less of this starch converted into readily absorbable sugars, your body simply can't access the calories it contains. It's like it doesn't even exist. In fact, this starch now acts more like fibre, not only promoting a greater feeling of fullness (despite containing less calories) but potentially even nourishing the friendly bacteria in your gut. Score!

A small clinical trial at the University of Toronto aimed to investigate this further by comparing the impact of cutting 500 calories from the daily diets of overweight people with simply adding the equivalent of 120g of mixed beans and lentils (about half a drained can) every day. The people in the bean group were free to continue eating whatever they wanted, just as long as they ate the extra beans, too, so in theory would be consuming a significantly greater number of calories. After 8 weeks *both* groups saw their waistlines shrink, their systolic blood pressure fall and their insulin sensitivity improve equally. But the bean eaters had a slight edge over the calorie counters, being the only group to see their levels of 'good' HDL cholesterol rise, as well as their fasting C peptide (a measure associated with reduced diabetes risk). Eat more and see your waistline shrink? Sounds good to me!

 ## THE BEST BEANS GOING ············

Most beans have similar levels of protein, fibre and minerals, but it's the levels of potentially heart-healthy polyphenols that set them apart. Pretty far apart, in some cases, according to a trial published by the United States Department of Agriculture, and depth of colour seems to be a pretty good indicator. The darker the bean, the greater the polyphenol punch, so choose wisely.

 ## SUPER SOYA

Soya is a bit of an exception when it comes to all other beans. Not only does it have twice as much protein gram for gram, but also, unlike pretty much any other plant food, this is a complete protein, containing significant amounts of all the amino acids needed by our bodies. This extra protein also means soya contains proportionally fewer carbs and therefore has significantly less impact on your blood sugar than regular beans (which already have a very low impact).

Compare them to an equal weight of steak, however, and they contain a third less protein. So why not just stick to meat? Well, a review that pooled the findings of 38 controlled clinical trials in humans concluded that 'the consumption of soy protein rather than animal protein significantly decreased serum concentrations of total cholesterol, ['bad'] LDL

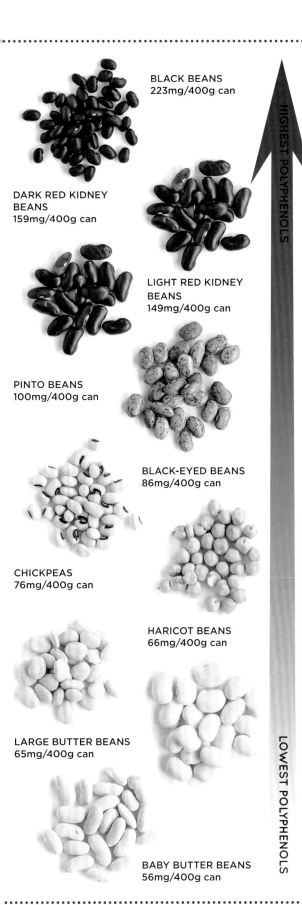

BLACK BEANS
223mg/400g can

DARK RED KIDNEY
BEANS
159mg/400g can

LIGHT RED KIDNEY
BEANS
149mg/400g can

PINTO BEANS
100mg/400g can

BLACK-EYED BEANS
86mg/400g can

CHICKPEAS
76mg/400g can

HARICOT BEANS
66mg/400g can

LARGE BUTTER BEANS
65mg/400g can

BABY BUTTER BEANS
56mg/400g can

HIGHEST POLYPHENOLS

LOWEST POLYPHENOLS

cholesterol, and triglycerides'. A pretty compelling reason to swap the odd burger for a bean version (such as my Ultimate Beet Burger on page 85).

PERFECT PLATE PARTNERS

All over the world beans are traditionally paired with rice, and stirring a can of these into your next pilaf could make a big difference to its health benefits according to a study published in the *Journal of Nutrition*. Researchers found that adding different types of beans to a white rice meal could consistently blunt the impact of carbohydrate on blood sugar for up to 3 hours after consumption. Out of the three bean varieties tested, black and pinto appeared to have a slight edge over kidney beans.

These results echo the findings of other studies, such as one that tracked the diets of Costa Ricans (who eat rice and beans together at almost every meal) and found that people who preferred a higher proportion of beans to rice consistently had lower blood pressure, levels of blood sugar and harmful fats. So much so in fact, the researchers concluded: 'Substituting one serving of beans for one serving of white rice was associated with a 35 per cent lower risk of metabolic syndrome or pre-diabetes.' Astonishingly, the blood-sugar-blunting effects of beans can even carry over to the next meal, reducing (albeit slightly) the impact of carb-heavy meals eaten several hours later and even the next day – a phenomenon known as the 'Second Meal Effect'. Looking for a recipe to combine the two? See page 180 for my Saffron Rice & Beans, which sneakily cuts the carbs and ups the protein with tasty black beans.

HOW TO EAT BEANS &
KEEP YOUR FRIENDS

Worried about the, ahem, 'after-effects' of bean consumption? According to a trial at Arizona State University up to 11 per cent of the time it's all in our heads. When given a placebo meal containing no flatulence-producing foods, when asked, a significant proportion of participants still reported getting terrible wind. The same trial also suggested that black-eyed beans produced less than half the windy effects of kidney or black beans. Want to do your best to keep your friends? The UK's National Health Service claims that there is some evidence that drinking peppermint or ginger tea can help improve the symptoms. Get the kettle on, quick!

OVEN-BAKED BEANS

Bung everything in a tray and be tucking in in about an hour. This stuff is almost as easy as opening a can, but so much tastier and better for you. Delicious served on wholegrain toast with poached eggs and fresh watercress.

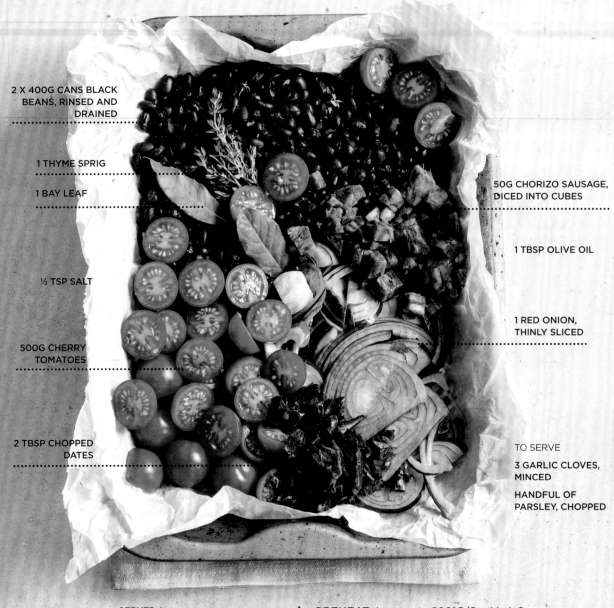

2 X 400G CANS BLACK BEANS, RINSED AND DRAINED

1 THYME SPRIG

1 BAY LEAF

½ TSP SALT

500G CHERRY TOMATOES

2 TBSP CHOPPED DATES

50G CHORIZO SAUSAGE, DICED INTO CUBES

1 TBSP OLIVE OIL

1 RED ONION, THINLY SLICED

TO SERVE

3 GARLIC CLOVES, MINCED

HANDFUL OF PARSLEY, CHOPPED

SERVES 4
PREP TIME 10 MINUTES
COOK TIME 50–65 MINUTES

PREHEAT the oven to 200°C/Gas Mark 6.

COMBINE all the ingredients except the garlic and parsley in a roasting tin and season well.

BAKE for 50–65 minutes, or until the sauce has thickened.

STIR through the garlic and parsley and serve.

EDAMAME GUACAMOLE

Teaming up the classic combination of beans and avocado cuts the fat and ups the protein in my quirky take on this Mexican favourite – serve with slices of toasted wholemeal pitta bread or with crudités, or both! More substantial and satisfying than the original, yet every bit as delicious. This even got the thumbs up from my Mexican buddy, Ruth. *Ay Madre*!

MAKES 200G

PREP TIME 10 MINUTES

....

100G COOKED EDAMAME BEANS, SHELLED

2 LARGE AVOCADOS, STONED, PEELED AND MASHED

FINELY GRATED ZEST OF ½ LIME

½ RED ONION, FINELY DICED

1 RED CHILLI, FINELY DICED

½ TSP SALT

BLITZ the cooked edamame beans in a food processor until you have a smooth purée, then scrape into a serving bowl.

MIX through the remaining ingredients and serve.

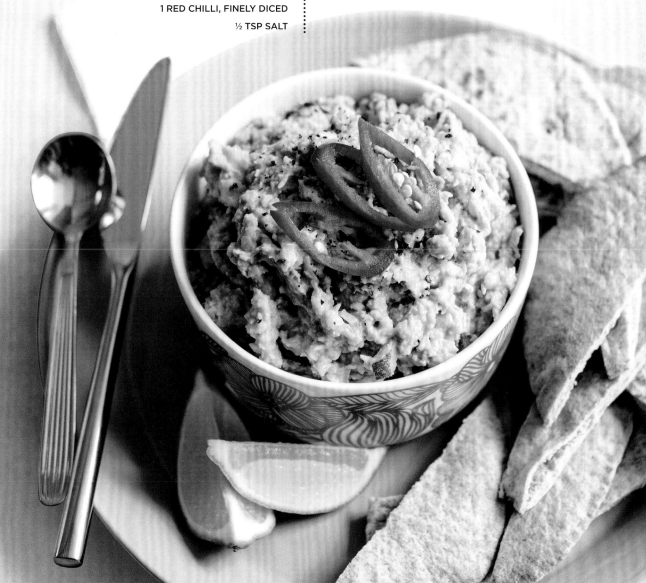

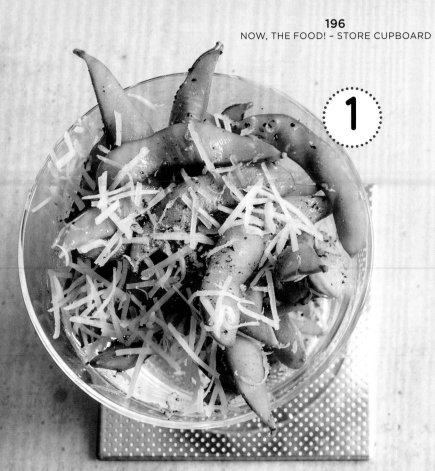

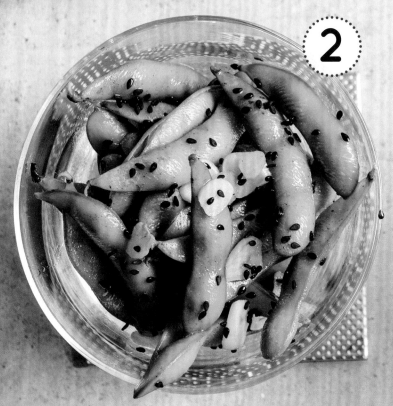

EDAMAME, THREE WAYS

Warm, satisfying and packed with protein, these green soya beans make a great starter or a side dish for any occasion. The beans are served in their pods; just bit into the pod and the bean pops into you both.

SERVES 2–4
PREP TIME 5 MINUTES
COOK TIME 3 MINUTES

450G FROZEN EDAMAME BEANS IN PODS
SALT

COOK the edamame beans in a saucepan of salted boiling water for 3 minutes, then drain.

HOW TO SERVE

1 LEMON, PARMESAN & PEPPER

Heat 1 tsp **olive oil** in a large frying pan, add the finely grated zest of 2 **lemons**, 1 tsp **black pepper** and the cooked **edamame beans** and toss until golden. Serve sprinkled with 50g grated **Parmesan cheese**.

2 SESAME & FLAKED GARLIC

Heat 1 tsp **olive oil** in a large frying pan, add 5 sliced **garlic cloves** and fry until golden and crisp. Add the cooked **edamame beans** and toss in the oil until golden. Serve sprinkled with toasted **sesame seeds**.

3 PAPRIKA & OLIVE OIL

Heat 1 tbsp **olive oil** in a large frying pan, add the cooked **edamame beans** and toss with 2 tsp **hot smoked paprika** until golden.

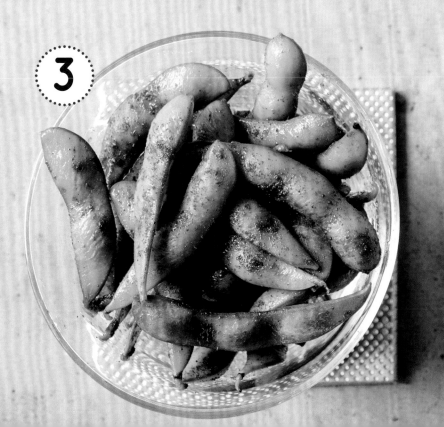

3

ROAST CHICKPEA CROUTONS

All the crunch of fresh-baked croutons, but with a much more satisfying protein.
As versatile as they are tasty, I love these in salads, atop soups, as a crisp garnish to
vegetable and rice dishes or even blended up to make a smoky, roasted hummus.

MAKES 800G
PREP TIME 5 MINUTES
COOK TIME 40 MINUTES

....

2 X 400G CANS CHICKPEAS, DRAINED AND RINSED
2 TBSP OLIVE OIL
1 TSP HOT SMOKED PAPRIKA
1 TSP GARLIC POWDER
½ TSP SALT

PREHEAT the oven to 200°C/Gas Mark 6.

PLACE all the ingredients in a large bowl and toss together, then tip into a large baking sheet.

ROAST for 40 minutes, or until the chickpeas are crisp and golden. Serve warm or cold.

STORE in an airtight container for up to 2 weeks.

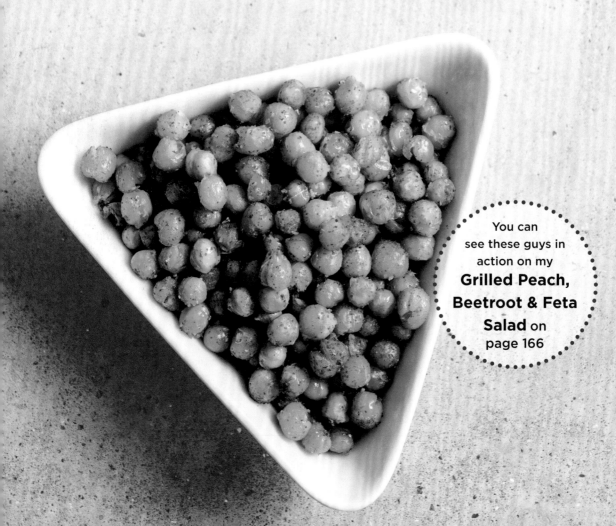

You can
see these guys in
action on my
**Grilled Peach,
Beetroot & Feta
Salad** on
page 166

HUMMUS

Homemade hummus is shockingly simple to make and with a flavour that is a world away from anything you can buy. The veggie-enhanced versions below are so packed with the good stuff, you won't even notice I have sneakily reduced the fat.

MAKES 800G

PREP TIME 10 MINUTES

....

2 X 400G CANS CHICKPEAS, DRAINED AND RINSED

2 TBSP TAHINI

2 GARLIC CLOVES, MINCED

1 TSP SALT

FINELY GRATED ZEST AND JUICE OF 1 LEMON

4 TBSP EXTRA VIRGIN OLIVE OIL

½ TSP PAPRIKA

PITTA BREAD OR CRUDITÉS, TO SERVE

BLITZ the chickpeas, tahini, garlic, salt and lemon zest and juice in a food processor until smooth. With the motor still running, gradually drizzle in the oil through the funnel until combined. You may need to stir in 2–3 tablespoons water to get it to the desired consistency.

SPOON into a serving bowl and sprinkle with the paprika. Serve with pitta or crudités.

VARIATIONS

1 AVOCADO

Add 1 stoned, peeled and roughly chopped **avocado** and make as above.

2 RED PEPPER

Add 3 **roasted red peppers** from a jar and make as above.

3 BEETROOT

Add 2 pre-cooked roughly chopped **cooked beetroot** and make as above.

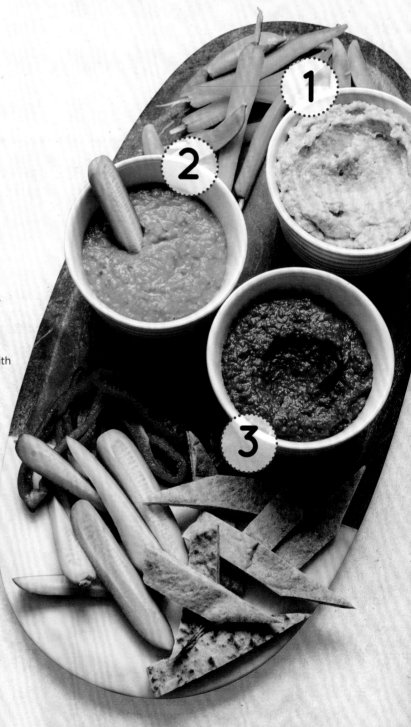

COFFEE

I couldn't live without coffee. But for years the drink has been considered an unhealthy vice by health-food warriors, who claim its 'toxic' caffeine is terrible for your heart and your mood, and even a potential cause of cancer. Thank goodness the evidence says quite the opposite! Let me explain...

In reality, coffee turns out to be an incredibly rich source of heart-healthy polyphenols, containing much more than fruit and veg like blackberries and even (gasp!) kale per serving. Indeed, your daily Americano actually boasts more than double the polyphenol content of a purist's green tea, plus a range of demonstrated health benefits. Coffee lovers, rejoice!

 ## SHARP MINDS, GOOD MOODS

Track the health of coffee drinkers versus non-coffee drinkers over up to 30 years and what do you find? Well, according to a paper in the journal *Clinical Nutrition* that pooled together the results of studies involving almost 35,000 participants, people drinking 1–2 cups of coffee a day experienced a significantly lower risk of developing cognitive disorders, including Alzheimer's disease and dementia.

This positive effect on mental health can also be seen in a much shorter timescale. Moderate doses of caffeine have been demonstrated to not only boost feelings of alertness, but also improve mood within minutes of consumption. This well-established effect appeared to be reflected in a study by the Harvard School of Public Health, which found that women who drank 2–3 cups of coffee a day were 15 per cent less likely to suffer from depression. Add a couple extra, upping the dose to 4 or more cups a day, and the risk was reduced up to 20 per cent. Why do we think it was the caffeine at work? Well, drinkers of decaf experienced no such benefit, with other reviews of studies measuring total caffeine consumption (in teas, coffees and other drinks) finding extremely similar results.

CARDIOVASCULAR HEALTH

The American Heart Association set a group of stats geeks to work trawling through dozens of studies on how coffee drinking affected the health of 1.3 million volunteers. Months of calculations later, they found that even at the highest coffee consumption of over 5 cups a day there was no negative effect on heart health. None. In fact, more moderate consumption was associated with a significant reduction in risk of heart disease, stroke and diabetes – by as much as 12–15 per cent. And in this case it didn't appear to be the caffeine at work, either, with decaf drinkers experiencing a similar benefit. The authors suggested it may be other natural-occurring chemicals in the coffee bean, such as the polyphenols, providing this apparent protective effect. Who funded this study? Nope, not some giant coffee chain, but the not-for-profit US National Institutes of Health.

 ## LOWER CANCER RISK?

According to the evidence we have so far, a regular coffee habit is not associated with an increase in cancer risk. In fact, in the case of colorectal, liver, breast and prostate cancers it appears it may even help reduce your risk. One review by the University of Southern California, for instance, reported that coffee drinking (both decaf and regular) was associated with a 26 per cent lower incidence of colorectal cancer versus non-drinkers. What's more, this reduction was found to be dose dependent, with the incidence of cancer falling steadily the more coffee people drank (from 22 per cent at 1 cup a day to 64 per cent at 3.5 cups or more). Such dose-dependent relationships suggest this association was not mere coincidence, and it was really the coffee itself that was behind this benefit.

 ## TOO MUCH OF A GOOD THING?

Of course, coffee consumption can also result in nervousness or disrupted sleep if drunk to excess or late at night. So don't go crazy. During pregnancy women are generally advised by public health bodies like the American College of Obstetricians and Gynecologists and the UK's National Health Service to halve their caffeine intake to a maximum of 200mg a day, which is roughly equivalent to 2 cups of coffee. Other than that, feel free to indulge in your (up to) '5-a-day'.

ROBUSTA IS RICHEST

Aside from caffeine, one of the key compounds researchers believe to be behind coffee's apparent health benefits is a group of compounds called chlorogenic acids. In fact, coffee is the richest of all food and drinks in this class of antioxidants, which contribute to the acidic notes in the drink. But not all coffee beans were made equal. Those from the *robusta* species contain twice as much chlorogenic acid and bitter-tasting caffeine than the more expensive *arabica* types. They also have a bolder flavour as a result. Although I generally recommend filter robusta coffee, as it's these cheaper beans that are often used to make instant coffee, even everyday granules can be higher in this class of phytonutrients than fancy ground arabica.

WHAT ABOUT DECAF?

Although part of coffee's health effects have been attributed to the very caffeine itself, if you are want to avoid the buzz, there is more good news. The decaffeination process apparently only destroys small amounts of chlorogenic acids (about 3–9 per cent) and has very little effect on coffee's total antioxidant activity. This may explain why some studies find that even decaf coffee drinkers experience many of its health benefits.

FILTER ALL THE WAY

According to the journal *Food Chemistry*, preparing coffee using the filter technique is by far the best way to extract the all-important polyphenols, containing 50 per cent more per serving than espresso, almost twice that of percolator and over three times that of instant.

Filter coffee also has the rather fortunate side-effect of straining out two other natural substances found in coffee beans called cafestol and kahweol, which some studies suggest may raise 'bad' LDL cholesterol. Percolated coffee and the industrial processes used to make instant coffee do a similar job. However, cafetiere, espresso and Turkish-style coffee contain relatively higher amounts, which might slightly raise cholesterol over time. So stick to filter if you can.

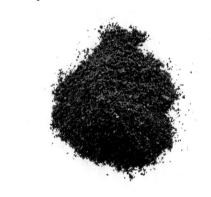

LIGHT ROASTING, HEAVY ANTIOXIDANTS

Sadly, the roasting process that gives coffee beans their characteristic caramel, nutty and smoky notes also destroys a large percentage of their heat-sensitive polyphenols. How much are we talking? Dark roasts can lose between 90 and 100 per cent of their chlorogenic acids as they tumble in the kiln – benefits potentially totally eliminated! Pick a medium roast, though, and you retain far more, with losses of around 70 per cent. Go for a light roast and about 50 per cent of the polyphenols remain intact. This means that choosing a pale roast can give you a polyphenol payload a whopping five times greater than a dark one – a simple swap that could make a big difference.

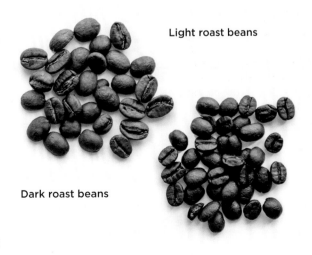

Light roast beans

Dark roast beans

TEA

Ask people to name a bunch of 'superfoods' and it's a fair bet that green tea will come out pretty close to the top of that list. Indeed, being one of the richest dietary sources of heart-healthy polyphenols, green tea is said to do everything from inducing rapid weight loss to helping stave off cancer. There is only one problem with many of these health claims, however: they just aren't supported by the evidence. As a total tea addict, I think this is big shame, as these claims deflect from the broad array of potential benefits that tea *does* offer, backed by more solid science and all for essentially zero calories. This section is dedicated to revealing tea truths and busting a few myths along the way, all to uncover how to get the very best out of your cuppa.

♡ CANCER PREVENTING? (ACTUALLY...MAYBE NOT)

In 2009, an independent, international team of experts sifted through the best available evidence to date, gathering together over 50 studies that involved a massive 1.6 million participants to see if they could find a consistent link between tea drinking and the incidence of a range of different cancers. After crunching the numbers, the researchers found paper after paper that strongly suggested tea consumption was indeed associated with a lowered risk of developing cancer. Many had been enthusiastically reported by the press, no doubt cementing green tea's 'superfood' status in the public imagination.

The tricky thing is, however, that these positive trials were also matched by scores of others that found the exact opposite, suggesting that tea drinking really had little or no protective effect, creating a body of highly contradictory evidence – notice how the press left out this little detail? With the exception of liver cancer (for which there was only one study), the evidence for all cancer types was so conflicting that no meaningful patterns could be identified. The authors concluded, pretty firmly, that 'There should be no expectation that drinking green tea regularly will reduce the risk of cancer.' Damn!

♡ FAT BURNING? (SORRY, NOT THIS EITHER)

The same reviewing body then turned its attentions to green tea and weight loss. Collating the findings of 18 of the best-quality studies from around the world that put tea drinking to the test on a total of nearly 2,000 overweight or obese volunteers, this time the researchers did find a positive effect. In fact, all the studies unanimously showed that participants lost more weight on average than those taking a placebo. Cue 'Weight-loss Wonder' headlines.

How much more weight did they lose? Well, after excluding studies with extremely outlying findings, the average total weight loss was about 600g per person – after 3 months of daily consumption. Hardly earth-shattering. In fact, in some trials this reduction was as low as a pitiful 20–100g. The killjoy scientists concluded that weight loss on this scale is so minor that it would have no meaningful effect on health (or, frankly, on your appearance). So, sadly, don't expect a matcha miracle.

♡ LOWER RISK OF HEART DISEASE

Now for some good news. Daily tea consumption has been consistently shown to be associated with lowered blood pressure and cholesterol levels (two key risk factors in developing heart disease and stroke) across at least a dozen studies. In fact, in a recent review that tracked the lifestyles of over 850,000 participants, researchers found that drinking just 375ml of tea a day (about one large mug) was associated with a 27 per cent lower risk of heart disease and an 18 per cent lower risk of stroke. This is believed to be a result of a group of antioxidant polyphenols in tea called catechins, which have potent anti-inflammatory effects.

The Journal of Clinical and Diagnostic Research reports that the **natural antibacterial compounds in green tea** make it **equally as effective as commercial mouthwash,** despite being cheaper and safe to swallow.

HIGHEST POLYPHENOLS

Up to

10x

the catechins of
black tea

LOWEST POLYPHENOLS

Green & white tea

Dry the fresh, young leaves of tea plants, and, hey presto, you have yourself green tea. This minimal processing has been shown by a stack of studies to retain the highest levels of their natural polyphenols – including the all-important catechins. In fact, according the University of Leeds, green varieties averaged out as containing almost *seven times* more catechins than ordinary 'builder's' types, rising up to tenfold when you compared the lowest black teas with the most potent greens.

It is often claimed that super-posh white tea, made from the very youngest tips, is even higher. However the evidence here isn't very clear. According to *Journal of Food Science*, for example, although the most potent whites could contain up to 60 per cent more catechins than the richest greens, in general there was a wide variation and a huge overlap in the phytonutrient content between these two groups.

Oolong tea

Never heard of this? Well, it is a sort of halfway house between exotic greens and traditional black teas. Here, the freshly picked leaves are slightly bruised to expose the compounds they contain to the air. This triggers the release of an enzyme called polyphenol oxidase, which causes the leaves to turn brown (just as happens when you cut or bruise an apple, see page 115). The result is a tea with a slightly more intense, subtle bitterness and darker colour. Polyphenol oxidase really does what it says on the tin. It *oxidizes* the polyphenols in the leaves, cancelling out some of their *anti*oxidant benefits, causing levels of catechins to dip. Darjeeling and 'Chinese restaurant' jasmine teas are classic examples of this type of tea. They are still much higher in catechins than the average black tea (60 per cent more, according to the University of Leeds team) but nowhere near a match for greens.

Black tea

Take the same semi-processed oolong-type teas and leave them for even longer, often at hot, humid temperatures, until they start to ferment, and this oxidation reaction goes into overdrive. For this reason black teas typically have much lower catechin levels and antioxidant activity, as well as the darkest colour and strongest flavour of them all. When the catechins in the leaves are fermented, they are turned into another group of substances called theaflavins (which are technically also polyphenols). Although some early test-tube studies have suggested these, too, may have beneficial effects, the evidence base is, so far, much less than that for the catechins found in green teas.

MATCHA TEA

Take dried green tea leaves and run them through a stone mill and you get one of the biggest food trends of recent years – matcha tea powder. Whisked into hot water to create a creamy, jade green concoction, this super-fancy tea sells in tiny packets in my local supermarket for an eye-watering 80 times the price of regular green types. So what's all the fuss about?

Well, according to the back of the packet of one brand, matcha contains 137 times the antioxidants of traditional types. And this may seem plausible, because whisked into a drink you are consuming every last bit of the tea leaf, not just the soaking water before the spent leaves have been chucked in the bin. This stat isn't made up, either – it's from a 2003 study at the Department of Chemistry, University of Colorado, that also found matcha contained at least three times those of the highest-ever published value in the literature for green tea. Hence the explosion of recipes for matcha lattes, smoothies and even cheesecake on wellness blogs. I mean, if it's emerald-coloured, exotic *and* expensive, it must be healthy. Right?

The problem is that one of the key hallmarks of a sound science is that it needs to be duplicable. If you repeat the same experiment, similar results should happen. But in the case of matcha, these miraculous levels just haven't been found by anyone else. In one study at the University of Bologna that investigated all sorts of green and white teas, for example, it was found that matcha's levels of catechins were very middle of the road, lower than jasmine and plain old Ceylon. These findings have been duplicated by at least two other Japanese studies, which showed several everyday green teas to contain far higher levels of catechins than matcha (despite a far more reasonable price tag).

STORAGE IS KEY

Even once dried, the process of natural oxidation continues in tea leaves, slowly reducing their antioxidant levels over time, according to a study by the United States Department of Agriculture. In the first-ever study to address the effect of storage on tea polyphenols, the US researchers found that after 6 months of storage at room temperature, the levels of some catechins could more than halve. There are three simple things you can do to avoid this happening: buy your tea in small batches and purchase a little more frequently (rather than purchasing in big packs that sit in your cupboard for months), and store it in a sealed container in a cool place to help slow down the reactions that can knock tea's phytonutrient content and flavour for six.

SWAP MILK FOR LEMON?

When you add a splash of milk to tea, the protein it contains binds to some of the bitter polyphenols, giving it a much smoother flavour. But for this very reason some scientists postulated that it may also impede tea's health benefits, and certainly, there is some limited evidence from two small trials that this may indeed be the case. Yet, as often happens in science, there are confusingly four other trials out there that found milk to have no such negative effect. The balance of evidence, therefore, seems to be tipping in milk's favour.

However, if you like your tea with lemon, you just might be on to a good thing. Two early studies have suggested that consuming tea with added vitamin C (such as that naturally found in lemons) may significantly improve the absorption of polyphenols. In fact, a little squirt of lemon could send the amount of bioavailable catechins soaring over five times, according to a test-tube study at Purdue University in the United States. Nothing 100 per cent conclusive, as yet, but a slice of lemon makes a tasty alternative way to serve your cuppa, and just might have a nutritional edge over milk.

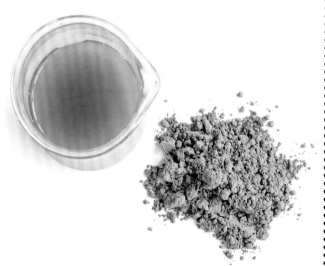

A squirt
of lemon might
make tea's catechins

5x

more
absorbable

♨ PREPARATION

How you make and serve tea is almost as important as variety choice in determining its polyphenol content. But this doesn't mean loads of fuss. Make a couple of small swaps here and you could get even more out of each cup.

Brew very hot...

Tea snobs will tell you that tea should never be made with boiling water, but with water heated to only 80°C. But what does the science say? Well, according to the University of Leeds (yes, them again), boiling-hot water straight from the kettle proved significantly more effective at drawing out the catechins from the tea leaves than water at 80°C. In fact, simply ignoring the tea aficionados' advice (how are you supposed to measure 80°C at home, anyway?) could reward you with over 50 per cent more of the good stuff. The same team also found that by leaving the bag in the water for 10 minutes (5 minutes longer than average), you could boost this by up to an extra 40 per cent.

Leaving your tea to brew for just a couple of extra minutes longer can mean other important benefits too. According to the International Agency for Research on Cancer, drinking very hot liquids of 65°C and over can double the risk of throat cancer over the long term. After just 6 minutes of brewing, however, the temperature of freshly brewed tea in a mug falls to well within the safe zone at 60°C according the Northumbria University – meaning the longer brew can be better for you in two different ways.

...or very cold

If high temperatures are more effective, it makes the new trend for cold-infused teas sound like a distinctly bad idea. Coming out of places like Taiwan in recent years, these methods involve soaking tea leaves in water at room temperature for at least 2 hours or in the fridge overnight to produce a refreshing, cold-brewed iced tea. This process is different from ordinary iced tea, which is just chilled hot-brewed tea, and is said to create a much more delicate, complex result.

Curious to find out more, a bunch of researchers at the University of Parma decided to put this to the test in a series of experiments. Making loads of varieties of tea from using both hot and cold treatments, they found the cold-brewing technique surprisingly extracted not only more catechins, but also more polyphenols overall, and had higher antioxidant activity. This is because although high temperatures are more effective at extracting polyphenols rapidly (in the 5 minutes you

normally brew tea for), they also destroy some of the polyphenols in the process. Making a refreshing iced tea using this long, slow steeping at low temperatures appears (in some varieties at least) to retain the maximum amount of polyphenols. It also happens to be the very easiest method. Just chuck some tea leaves (or bags) in a jug of water, pop it in the fridge overnight and you are done.

According to the Parma team, there seemed to be a difference between varieties, too, with green and black teas brewed in this way having over 40 per cent more polyphenols – with oolong containing even more, showing a significant 64 per cent boost. One study at the University of Bologna found that white tea was one of the very best candidates for this cold treatment, containing around twice the catechins when steeped cold. While not all research has shown this boosting effect in the steeping of every variety, all show cold-brewing to be roughly comparable if not better. Not bad, considering it takes less work and energy.

TEA & HYDRATION

Extremely low in calories yet high in phytonutrients, tea might seem like a great way to keep yourself hydrated, whether it's a chilled glass of iced tea in the summer or a warming cuppa at work. But does the caffeine it contains offset its benefits? A trial published in the *British Journal of Nutrition* decided to put this common claim to the test by giving a group of participants either 6 cups of black tea a day or an equal quantity of plain water, then measuring their blood and urine levels at continuous intervals. The researchers concluded that both tea and water were equally effective at hydration. A great option therefore for people who want something a bit more interesting than tap without the sugar rush of squash or juice.

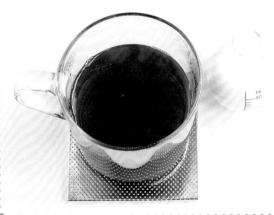

JASMINE CHICKEN WITH GREEN TEA NOODLES

Tea and chicken soup don't sound like they would work together, but boy they do. The delicate fragrance and pleasant bitterness of tea adds an extra complexity to comforting chicken broth, while at the same time boosting its polyphenol content. Yum!

SERVES 4

PREP TIME 10 MINUTES, PLUS INFUSING

COOK TIME ABOUT 15 MINUTES

3 TBSP LOOSE-LEAF GREEN TEA

1.5 LITRES BOILING WATER

4 BONELESS, SKINLESS CHICKEN BREASTS, ABOUT 100G EACH

3 CHICKEN OR VEGETABLE STOCK CUBES, CRUMBLED

50G SLICED DRIED SHIITAKE MUSHROOMS

2 CARROTS , CUT INTO MATCHSTICKS

1 THUMB-SIZED PIECE OF FRESH ROOT GINGER, PEELED AND CUT INTO MATCHSTICKS

3 GARLIC CLOVES, MINCED, PLUS 2 GARLIC CLOVES, SLICED

500G GREEN TEA SOBA NOODLES

4 SPRING ONIONS, SLICED

50ML CHINESE RICE WINE OR SHERRY

1 TSP SESAME OIL

2 SMALL RED CHILLIES, THINLY SLICED

1 TSP SESAME SEEDS

PUT the tea leaves in a large, heatproof jug and pour over the boiling water. Cover and leave to infuse for 10 minutes.

STRAIN the tea into a large, shallow saucepan and bring to a simmer over a medium-high heat. Add the chicken, stock cubes, mushrooms, carrots, ginger and minced garlic and simmer for 10–15 minutes, or until the chicken is cooked through.

MEANWHILE, cook the noodles according to the packet instructions.

REMOVE the vegetables and chicken from the broth using a slotted spoon, then slice the chicken into pieces.

DIVIDE the cooked soba noodles between 4 bowls and pour over the hot broth.

ARRANGE the chicken and vegetables over the top, then sprinkle with the spring onions, chillies, sliced garlic, sesame seeds, rice wine or sherry, sesame oil.

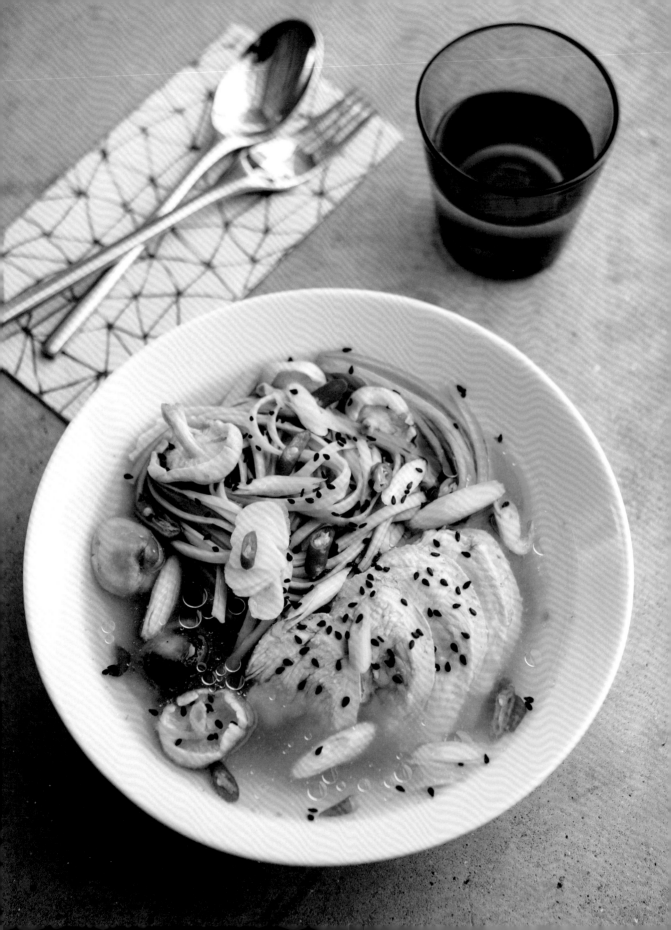

CHOCOLATE

From healthy-eater's pariah to nutritional powerhouse, chocolate's foodie reputation has experienced quite a turnaround in just two short decades, at least when it comes to the dark stuff. It is, after all, packed with loads of essential minerals, boasting significantly more iron, magnesium, potassium and zinc than even the almighty kale, gram for gram. Not to mention a host of antioxidant polyphenols, which evidence suggests may have heart-healthy effects. So it's not surprising that the press likes to proclaim the amazing 'superfood' benefits of chocolate as the latest good news story. But now for some context...

Chocolate is indeed very rich in minerals gram for gram, but it is also monumentally high in fat and sugar, which gives it ten times the calories of kale, so chocolate versus kale isn't really the greatest comparison. Calorie for calorie, in the health-benefit stakes, almost all fruit and veg beat chocolate hands down. And when you look at the scientific evidence behind the frequently reported health benefits of chocolate, such as improved mood, lowering of blood pressure and a boost to memory, well, there really aren't that many well-conducted trials out there that actually back this up.

Digging through the data, however, it turns out there are some areas where the research does look very promising, and compared to other sweet treats chocolate stills pack a hefty polyphenol punch. The best news is, there are simple, yet tasty ways to maximize the flavour and potential benefits in each calorie of this melt-in-the mouth deliciousness. Here's how to make chocolate even better.

♡ CIRCULATORY BENEFITS?

One of the most popular claims about chocolate is that it is good for heart health. However, its impact on common measures like blood pressure, for example, appear to be minor and, frankly, pretty inconsistent. Across the board I found 8 studies that showed a slight decrease in blood pressure; however, many more showed either no change (13 trials) or even a temporary *increase* (2 trials), which was attributed to chocolate's caffeine content – not exactly earth-shattering evidence.

However, there is some good news, particularly regarding circulation. As we age our arteries start to stiffen, impairing the circulation of blood around the body. As foods high in polyphenols have been reported to help combat this decline, a team at Yale University decided to put it to the test. They gave people a daily dose of hot cocoa for 6 weeks and found that this short intervention significantly improved the elasticity of their arteries, along with other measures of heart disease risk, without causing weight gain. And this wasn't a one-off either. Scores of studies from all over the world have reflected similar findings, and although there are exceptions, most seem to be in agreement. It is thought that a polyphenol called epicatechin found in particularly high levels in cocoa beans may be behind this effect. There is also some reasonable evidence to suggest that chocolate may also slightly reduce 'bad' LDL cholesterol, without affecting 'good' HDL or overall cholesterol levels, according to a review in the *European Journal of Clinical Nutrition*. Pass the hot cocoa!

♡ BRAIN FUNCTION? (PROBABLY NOT)

What could improved circulation mean for the rest of the body? Well, getting more blood flow to the brain, for example, *theoretically* might improve mental function. And certainly, when researchers at the University of Lisbon looked into the diets of older people, they did indeed find that those who happened to eat more chocolate seemed to also have significantly reduced risk of cognitive decline. But is this just a random coincidence? Well, what makes this intriguing is that in other studies the polyphenols in chocolate have also been shown to cross into the brain itself and accumulate in regions associated with learning and memory.

So what happened when researchers actually fed people dark chocolate and systematically measured their brain power? A team at Swinburne University in Australia gave middle-aged men and women a daily chocolate drink, rich in polyphenols, for a month. The University of Nottingham gave young female students a dose of cocoa every day for 5 days. Virginia State University gave a bunch of elderly people a plain old bar of dark chocolate a day for 6 weeks. And guess what they all found? Zero improvement in tests of mental function in all studies. When it comes to the claims of brain health, evidence here seems less promising, for now at least.

♡ SKIN AGEING

So here's a weird one. A small range of studies suggests that the polyphenols in chocolate may help prevent the damage to skin caused by UV light, which is thought to be one of the leading causes of wrinkles. In one small study published in the *Journal of Nutrition*, daily cocoa consumption (cocoa powder mixed into a drink) was associated with a 15 per cent reduction in UV-induced skin damage after 6 weeks. Consume the drink for 3 months and the trial suggests this protection ramps up as high as 25 per cent, improving skin circulation and 'cosmetically relevant skin surface and hydration variables', too (lab geeks have such a way with words).

Keen to see if these findings were repeatable (the hallmark of good science), a slightly larger Korean trial gave women a similar high-polyphenol cocoa drink every day. After 6 months, tests revealed that the participants had measurably smoother skin, with improved elasticity and which was better protected against UV light. Before you bin the sunscreen it is important to note that a third trial at the University of Quebec didn't report any protective effects against UV, but did show a slight improvement in facial skin elasticity after adding just 30g of the sweet stuff to women's daily diet.

⛁ TOP OF THE CHOCS

One of the reasons why the science behind chocolate's health benefits seems so variable could well be because the amount fed to people in these studies differed enormously – as much as three times, from a few squares to well over a whole bar every day. Many of the studies with the most impressive results didn't even use actual chocolate at all, but plain cocoa powder, which has a very different chemical make-up. To make matters more confusing, the *type* of chocolate makes a huge difference, too. Even among different bars of dark chocolate, one University of Leeds study found a pretty astonishing ninefold difference in the levels of the polyphenol epicatechin.

Knowing the right form (and getting the correct dose) of chocolate can mean the difference between a potential health benefit or just scoffing a block of sweetened, saturated fat. Here's how it breaks down.

> Calorie for calorie, **cocoa powder** offers
>
> # 4x
>
> the polyphenols of the darkest **dark chocolate**

⛁ COCOA POWDER

Cocoa beans are made up of about 50 per cent fat, which is used to fuel the growth of the young seedling. The 50 per cent that's left is a bitter, dark brown powder crammed with biologically active chemicals produced by the plant to defend its seeds against infection and protect the fat in it from going rancid: cocoa powder.

As pretty much all the polyphenols and minerals are found here, going straight to the source instantly bypasses a colossal amount of fat and sugar, giving you the most concentrated possible dose of the good stuff. In fact, gram for gram, cocoa powder is the fourth-most polyphenol-rich ingredient of all foods tested so far, right behind star anise, peppermint and cloves (which we eat in much lower amounts).

Being packed full of flavour, but with far fewer calories, it means you can make super-chocolatey puddings, milkshakes and hot cocoa without piling on the pounds. With just 4 tablespoons of natural cocoa powder giving you the same amount of polyphenols and minerals as an 85g bar of dark chocolate, a single cup of comforting hot cocoa made using this could give you the beneficial amount for fewer than 250 calories, about half those of eating dark chocolate! There's more good news, too: cocoa powder is roughly a third fibre, so this same quantity gives you as much fibre as a serving of bran cereal, and swaps the torture of eating flakes of cardboard for the richest, thickest hot chocolate ever. Want a recipe? Have five, each in a deliciously different flavour (see page 211).

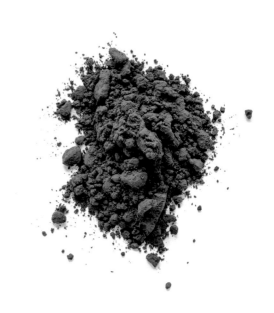

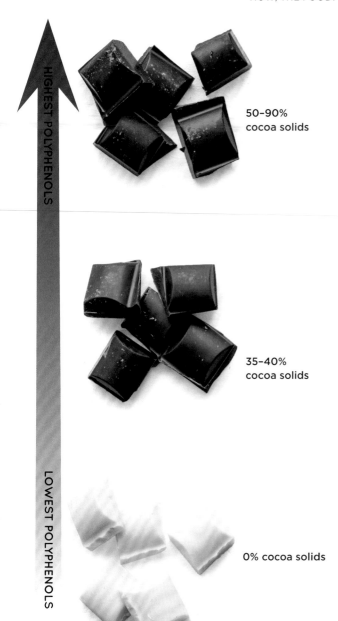

HIGHEST POLYPHENOLS

50–90%
cocoa solids

35–40%
cocoa solids

LOWEST POLYPHENOLS

0% cocoa solids

Dark chocolate

Dark chocolate takes the polyphenol-packed cocoa powder and dilutes it by adding back some of the creamy, fat-rich cocoa butter from the beans and sweetening it with sugar. Sadly, of course, this significantly waters down the powder's beneficial compounds with a tonne of extra calories. As it really only contains two ingredients – cocoa beans and sugar – the percentage of cocoa solids on the label gives you an instant guide to how much sugar is in it. A 70 per cent bar contains about 30 per cent sugar, a 60 per cent bar about 40 per cent sugar, and so on.

Bottom line? The higher the cocoa solids, the more healthy polyphenols (and the less super-calorific sugars) you get, but none is a match for pure cocoa powder. According to the latest review of the evidence behind chocolate's health effects you'd need to eat between 50–200g a day to get the 100mg epicatechin that is thought to reliably improve circulation. That amounts to between 300 and 1,000 calories every day – the latter being roughly half your daily calorie dose in one go! Sadly, if we are talking heart health, it really is a case of go as dark as you dare – at least 85 per cent – or don't bother.

Milk chocolate

Milk chocolate is basically dark chocolate diluted again by adding loads of powdered milk to achieve a mix that is roughly equal parts sugar, milk and cocoa solids. With 80 per cent fewer polyphenols than dark, you'd need to eat 700g a day just to get enough epicatechin. That's a shocking 3,745 calories worth, some one and a half times the total number of calories you should eat a day.

White chocolate

The white stuff dispenses with cocoa powder altogether and just mixes cocoa butter with milk and sugar (and maybe a touch of vanilla, too). It's chemically akin to mixing butter and sugar together, e.g. buttercream icing, and contains zero polyphenols.

THE HEALTHIEST CHOCOLATE GOING

Want to cram more good stuff into the same number of calories, as if by magic? There is a simple solution. Just pick *sugar-free* dark chocolate. Now, I'm such a chocolate snob I used to shudder at the very thought of it, but I have to say I am genuinely surprised at how amazingly identical the stuff tastes. In this chocolate, sugar is replaced with alternative, naturally occurring sweeteners like maltitol, which provide about half the calories and affect your blood sugar far less. Pick a brand sweetened with inulin, a sugary-tasting, gel-like substance found in the roots of the chicory plant, and each square could contain up to 35 per cent prebiotic fibre and boost the levels of friendly bacteria in your gut. Less sugar, fewer calories, more fibre *and* the same great taste – why on earth not?

HOT CHOCOLATE

Smooth, rich and with a hefty polyphenol punch, each serving of this sugar-free hot cocoa offers up the phytonutrients and minerals of a 85g slab of dark chocolate, all for 50 per cent fewer calories.

MAKES 1 LARGE MUG
PREP TIME 5 MINUTES
COOK TIME 5 MINUTES

....

4 TBSP NATURAL COCOA POWDER (NON-DUTCHED, SEE PAGE 212)

1 TBSP GRANULATED STEVIA (BAKING BLEND)

1 TSP VANILLA EXTRACT

½ TSP MIXED SPICE

PINCH OF SALT

350ML SEMI-SKIMMED MILK

COMBINE the cocoa powder, stevia, vanilla extract, mixed spice and salt with a little of the milk in a large microwavable mug to make a smooth paste (this is a lot of cocoa, so this can take a while!), then gradually whisk in enough of the remaining milk to fill the mug.

HEAT in the microwave on high for 2–3 minutes. Done!

VARIATIONS

1 ORANGE ZEST

Make the hot chocolate as above, adding the finely grated zest of 1 **orange** to the ingredients. Top each mug with 1 tsp whipped **double cream**, a **dried orange slice** and a few **chocolate chips**.

2 SAFFRON

Crumble ½ tsp **saffron threads** into powder over a plate. Make the hot chocolate as above, adding the powdered saffron to the ingredients. Top each mug with 1 tsp whipped **double cream** and a few extra **saffron threads**.

3 MEXICAN SPICE

Make the hot chocolate as above, adding ¼ tsp **chilli powder** to the ingredients. Top each mug with 1 tsp whipped **double cream**, a small slice of **red chilli**, a sprinkling of **pink peppercorns** and add a **cinnamon stick** for stirring.

4 RED VELVET

Make the hot chocolate as above, replacing half of the milk with **beetroot juice**. (I know this sounds weird but it totally works, just like chocolate beetroot cake does.) Top each mug with 1 tsp whipped **double cream** and some **freeze-dried strawberries**.

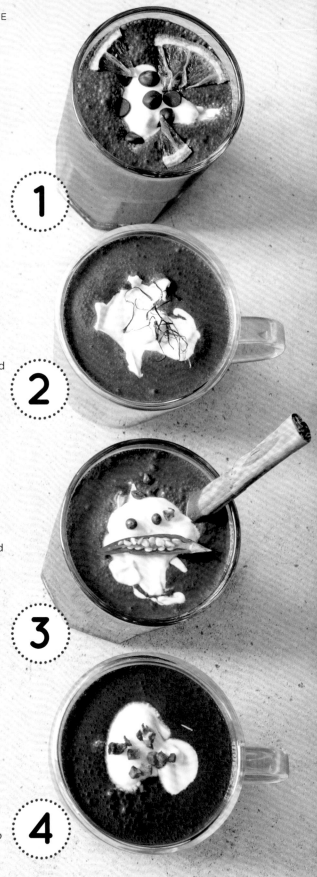

CHOCOLATE-HAZELNUT SPREAD

The stuff of childhood dreams, this healthier, homespun version is so packed full of polyphenol-rich dark cocoa powder and roasted hazelnuts there is no room left for added sugar or oil. It might have 70 per cent fewer calories than the shop-bought stuff, but you'd never know by its taste and texture.

Enjoying it as a treat with a big bowl of fresh fruit, instead of slathering it on sliced white, is a simple way to dramatically reduce the calories while upping the nutrition per serving at the same time. As always with chocolate, this concoction might be crammed full of good stuff but is still super-calorie dense, so go easy!

MAKES 400G

PREP TIME 15 MINUTES, PLUS COOLING

COOK TIME 5 MINUTES

....

150ML MILK

100G CHOPPED HAZELNUTS

2 TSP VANILLA EXTRACT

100G COCOA POWDER (NON-DUTCHED)

5 TBSP GRANULATED STEVIA (BAKING BLEND)

⅛ TSP SALT

POUR the milk and hazelnuts into a small saucepan and heat gently until the milk reaches simmering point. Remove from the heat, cover and leave to cool.

TRANSFER the nut and milk mixture to a food processor and blitz until as smooth as possible. This will take a good minute or two.

PUT the nut purée in a small bowl and fold in the remaining ingredients – at first it will seem like there isn't enough liquid, but it will get there.

STORE the mixture in a sterilized jar in a cool place (not the fridge) for up to 1 week. The spread will thicken on cooling.

'DUTCHED' SPELLS DISASTER

Potassium carbonate is a food additive used in some cocoa powders to balance out their acidity in a technique called 'dutching' or 'alkali treatment'. This chemical process can, however, slash its levels of heart-healthy polyphenols by more than 80 per cent. This is done by even the most fancy organic brands, and has in fact been used by chocolatiers for 180 years, so it might just be worth looking out for words 'potassium carbonate' on the ingredients label.

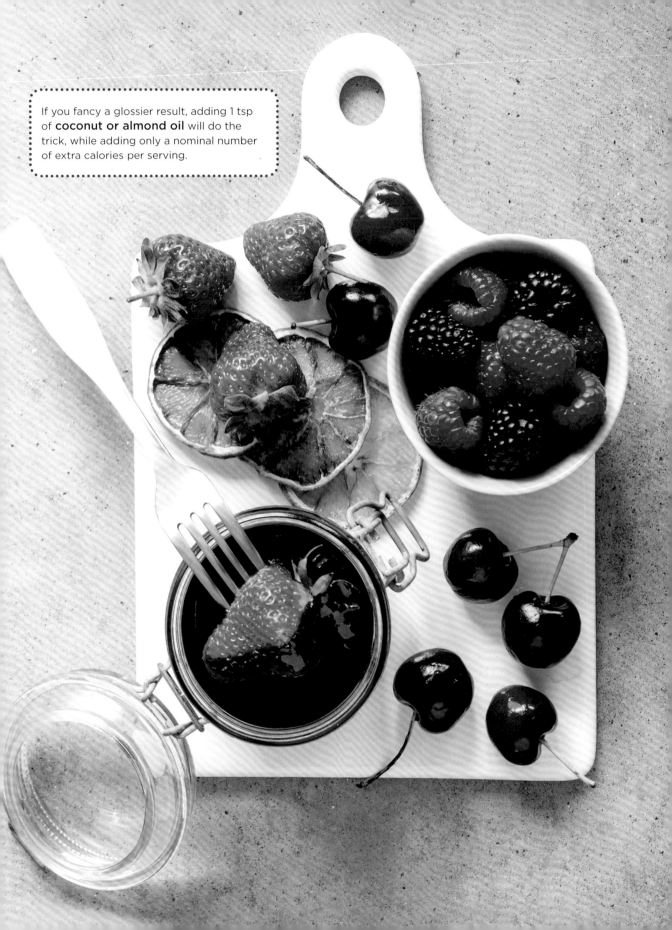

If you fancy a glossier result, adding 1 tsp of **coconut or almond oil** will do the trick, while adding only a nominal number of extra calories per serving.

BOOZE

We all know that drinking to excess is a bad idea, but could moderate alcohol consumption not only be safe, but actually *beneficial* to health? Well, a growing stack of observational studies suggests that a tipple or two a day might do just that. From heart disease and diabetes to certain types of stroke and even dementia, it appears that what at high doses is a poison, at low doses might indeed confer some protection. For those out there who, like me, enjoy a 'medicinal' glass or two with dinner, this section is dedicated to revealing the latest, most solid science on how to enjoy alcohol safely and potentially even healthily. Cheers!

♡ HEART PROTECTION

In one of the most comprehensive reviews ever, published in *The British Medical Journal*, researchers sifted through thousands of trials conducted over 50 years and selected the very best-quality studies, covering over a million participants. When they crunched the numbers, they found a consistent pattern emerging, showing that people who tended to have 1–2 alcoholic drinks a day also happened to have a 25 per cent reduced risk of heart disease. But was this just a random statistical coincidence? Well, the same team also found a strong association with this moderate level of alcohol consumption and significantly higher levels of 'good' HDL cholesterol. As this is linked to a reduced risk of developing heart disease, it also offers a plausible mechanism by which moderate drinking might improve heart health, suggesting that there was indeed a real connection.

However, even the most meticulously designed observational studies all share the same Achilles heel: they can never really prove a direct cause-and-effect relationship between the factors they observe, just an association, no matter how consistent their findings. For that you need a large clinical trial, which seeks out loads of resolute non-drinkers, gives them an identical, small dose of booze every day and then tracks the effect of this over a significant length of time. Perhaps surprisingly, scientists have simply never run such a trial...until now. Two brand-new Israeli studies took hundreds of teetotallers and gave them a small glass of wine (about 150ml) every day with dinner for up to 2 years. And guess what they found? In an almost perfect echoing of the observational studies, the Israeli teams reported that those drinking wine, particularly the red wine, showed significantly higher 'good' HDL cholesterol. The authors concluded that consumption at this level not only appears to be safe, it also may modestly reduce the risk of developing heart disease. It's very early days still, but a promising start!

♡ EYES, BONES, BRAINS & MORE

While most research has looked at the potential link between alcohol consumption and cardiovascular health, moderate drinking also appears to have a beneficial impact on an array of other conditions. For example, one large review by Loyola University Chicago found a 23 per cent reduced risk of Alzheimer's disease and other forms of dementia. For type 2 diabetes, a whole series of different reviews found up to a 30 per cent lower risk in moderate drinkers, with research also showing the risk of age-related bone-density loss to be significantly reduced among this group. One large Icelandic study even found a whopping 50 per cent reduction in the incidence of cataracts in older people who drank moderately versus total abstainers. Some pretty impressive stats! OK, so not as impressive as the kind of benefits you might see from, say, eating more fruit and veg or taking up regular exercise, but a nice thought that a glass of wine with dinner might well be doing you some good.

Moderate drinking could reduce the risk of heart disease by

25%

CREATIVITY BOOST?

It's not often you find a scientific study with a quirky title, so when I was trawling through the hundreds of papers on the effect of alcohol on health one called 'Uncorking the muse: alcohol intoxication facilitates creative problem-solving' really stood out. Published by the University of Illinois at Chicago, researchers set out to test the popular assumption that a glass or two of booze could boost creativity by getting college students tipsy and making them play word association games. No, really. Designed to test creative problem-solving abilities, these games proved significantly easier for those given either 2 pints of beer or 2 glasses of wine beforehand. The tipsy participants consistently outperformed a control group of those who were stone-cold sober; in fact, they delivered not only more correct answers, but also in a faster time.

But before you go downing shots before your next exam, the researchers also reported that this worked because it ironically reduced the participants' ability to concentrate, making them worse at completing problems that required attention control. Heightening one ability seemed to be caused by suppressing another. According to the team, being too focused can 'blind you to novel possibilities', claiming that 'sometimes it is good to be distracted'. Amen to that!

A SOBERING THOUGHT

Up the dose from 1–2 drinks a day to 3–4 drinks a day, however, and the same studies to show the benefits of moderate drinking *all* show them quickly evaporate. In fact, drinking more than a very moderate amount usually has the exact opposite effect, sending the risk of the same diseases alcohol may prevent in low doses soaring in higher doses, along with the risk of a whole range of cancers. In fact, in the particular case of breast, throat and mouth cancers, any level of alcohol consumption has been associated with a slight increase in risk, something that is particularly worth bearing in mind if you have these in your family history. On balance, however, the research so far does suggest that moderate drinking (i.e. no more than 2 glasses a day) does indeed have potential health benefits to most of the population, as long it is kept within these strict limits.

WHAT'S YOUR POISON?

OK, so alcohol may possess health benefits, but does the form in which you consume it – in wine, beer or spirits – make a difference? Well, most (but by no means all) studies do indeed suggest that wine drinkers have a slight edge over those who prefer beers and spirits. In one study at Holland's National Institute for Public Health and the Environment, for example, researchers found that while long-term light alcohol intake in general could reduce risk of death from heart diseases by almost a third, those drinking wine had marginally even better odds – including having a life expectancy up to 5 years longer than teetotallers. This frequently reported extra protective benefit of wine has been attributed to its higher levels of antioxidant polyphenols, which are significantly greater than those of beer, and almost nonexistent in highly distilled spirits like vodka.

In fact, in the Spanish Mediterranean diet – long considered a model for optimum health – wine and beer alone contribute a fifth of the total dietary antioxidants (16 per cent wine, 3 per cent beer). Some research, such as the Harvard Women's Health Study, has even suggested that while any level of general drinking may slightly raise breast cancer risk, when you specifically look at those who drink mainly red wine, this elevated risk is either reduced or even nonexistent.

While many of these studies also noted that this apparent extra benefit of wine might have more to do with other lifestyle factors in wine drinkers (such as lower smoking rates, higher fruit and veg consumption and lower saturated fat intake), getting a dose of extra polyphenols along with your daily tipple can't be a bad thing.

ONE-FIFTH

of the antioxidants in the Mediterranean diet come from **beer and wine**

🧺 WINE: RED BEATS WHITE

You've undoubtedly heard it before: red wine contains more of the good stuff than white. But how much more? Well, when it comes to heart-healthy polyphenols an astonishing ten times more than both white and paler rosé types, according to Clermont University in France. As the majority of the polyphenols in wine come from the red and purple pigments called anthocyanins, which give the grapes they are made from their characteristic hue, even amongst red wines, this furnishes us a wonderfully simple, colour-coded guide to which are likely to be the richest in phytonutrients.

LIGHT & FRESH

Grenache , Pinot Noir
Beaujolais

The lightest red wines tend to be made from grape varieties with thinner skins. This makes sense as the vast majority of the anthocyanin pigments in grapes are concentrated in the skin. The most common of them all is Pinot Noir, with its almost totally transparent pale colour. In one trial of 73 red wines by the University of São Paulo in Brazil, Pinot Noir was consistently the lowest of all varieties tested, containing a third less antioxidant activity than darker varieties like Syrah, Cabernet and Merlot.

MEDIUM

Malbec , Zinfandel
Cabernet Franc

Medium-bodied wines not only have a darker colour, but also a bolder, more gutsy flavour, which is caused by astringent chemicals called tannins that leach out of the grapes' skins and seeds. Tannins also happen to be polyphenols, meaning you get a double whammy of phytonutrients. This group of paler-coloured types includes the crowd-pleasers Malbec and Zinfandel, which lie at the darker end of the scale, right down to the paler Cabernet Franc.

DARK & FULL

Tannat , Pinotage , Syrah, Shiraz,
Cabernet Sauvignon, Merlot

The very darkest red wines are made from thick-skinned grape varieties. Winemakers often also leave them to soak for extra time after mashing to allow the maximum amount of colour and tannins to leach out. These wines have the boldest flavour, the fullest body and highest polyphenol content. It doesn't get any better than these.

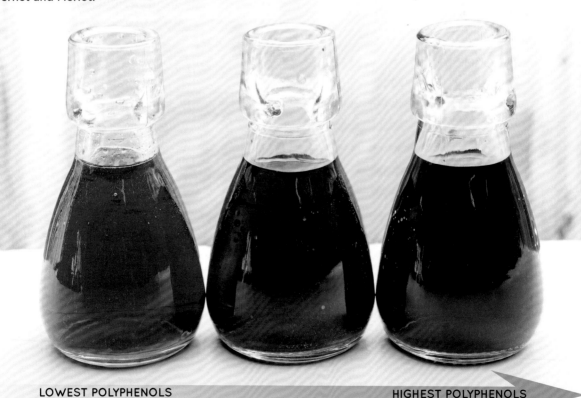

LOWEST POLYPHENOLS   HIGHEST POLYPHENOLS ➤

SEEK OUT THE SUNSHINE

Grapes are triggered to produce anthocyanins as a chemical defence against solar radiation, with the compounds acting as a sort of natural sunscreen to protect their cells against UV damage. In fact, trials have consistently shown that grapes grown in the shade can have up to 75 per cent fewer antioxidants. This also means that vines grown in hot, sunny climates tend to produce more anthocyanins – because of the extra sunshine and the lower rainfall, which helps further concentrate the compounds in the fruit. Pick the exact same variety grown in a cool region and you are likely to get less of the anthocyanin benefit. Here's a rough guide to how the regions break down.

Cool regions

Tasmania

New Zealand

Chile

Northern California and East Coast USA

Northern Europe

Hot regions

Argentina

Southern California

South Africa

Southern Europe

Australia

 ## PICK THEM YOUNG

During maturation and ageing, the original anthocyanin content of red wine continually declines, especially during the first 2 years after harvest. This is because these purple pigments are relatively unstable and slowly react with the tannins in the wine to form more stable related compounds called pyranoanthocyanins, which have a rusty, brownish colour.

It's this reduction in anthocyanins that gives aged wines their characteristic brick-red, as opposed to dark burgundy, colour, with the dwindling tannin levels resulting in a smoother, less astringent flavour that many people prefer. This means that despite retaining an overall red appearance, a significant proportion of the original anthocyanins in young red wine may be lost completely after a relatively short period of ageing. In one Czech study, for example, even deep red wine varieties like Merlot and Cabernet Sauvignon could lose around 30 per cent of their original anthocyanins within the first year of ageing alone. Tasty as it may be, reducing the levels of the very two groups of chemicals thought to be behind many of wine's health benefits isn't possibly the greatest idea. Plus younger wines are cheaper too!

A study of dozens of red wines by the University of São Paulo **found no correlation between price and antioxidant activity**. Yeh!

The **TANNAT GRAPE** has far higher levels of anthocyanins than most other red wines, with **45%** more than even deep, dark **Syrah** and up to **55%** more than rich reds like **Cabernet Sauvignon and Merlot**

🧺 BEER: SWITCH TO THE DARK SIDE

Like wine, the unique blend of phytonutrients in beer is believed to confer it extra benefits on top of just its alcohol content alone. Unlike the purple anthocyanins in wine grapes, however, these come from the complex mixture of dark-coloured compounds found mainly in the outer layers of malted barley grains, which contribute about 70 per cent of the polyphenols.

Indeed, according to the University of Valencia, the polyphenol content of beer is closely linked to its colour. This is partially due to the presence of a group of caramel-coloured polyphenols called proanthocyanidins, which make up the vast majority of polyphenols in the malt, where they contribute towards the final colour of the drink. Pick a dark malt beer and you could get nearly twice the polyphenols of paler lagers and as much as three times that of non-alcoholic lagers, which have some of their polyphenols removed at the same time as the booze.

When malt is toasted to make beer, another group of antioxidants called melanoidins are created. These are the brown pigments that are responsible for the colour of coffee, bread crust and chocolate, which add not only toasted flavour, but also potential health benefits – and of course make the beer even darker. Although these compounds aren't well absorbed by the body, they may be fermented by friendly bacteria in the gut to produce antioxidant compounds that *can* be absorbed by the body. Good to know my gut bacteria like beer as much as I do.

🧺 HOP UP THE BENEFITS

One of the reasons why dark beers tend to have such high polyphenol levels is that they tend to contain more added hops. These dried cones harvested from a climbing plant in the cannabis family are traditionally used to impart flavour and preserve the beer. While they might be added in tiny proportions, as little as 100 times less than those of malt, hops are so high in polyphenols that they contribute a third of the total content in many beers. In fact, it is these very polyphenols that are responsible for the plant's flavour-enhancing and preservative effects. Hops also help create the characteristic 'haze' of beers like ales, making them appear darker and denser than clear lagers. In short, the more bitter, cloudy and dark your pint, the more hop polyphenols your pint is likely to have.

BEER + BBQ = BEST FRIENDS

Beer and wine have been used as marinades to impart flavour to meat since ancient times. A whole range of recent scientific studies has also shown that this process can dramatically reduce the formation of potentially carcinogenic compounds called heterocyclic amines, which are formed when meat is cooked at high temperatures. But which is better? One study at Portugal's University of Porto put this to this test, comparing pan-fried beef marinated for 6 hours either in red wine or beer. The winner was the beer-based marinade, which not only slashed the production of these carcinogens by 88 per cent (more than twice that of red wine, which only reduced these 40 per cent), but was also considered to have a superior flavour in taste tests. In another trial, the same team also found that charcoal-grilled pork marinated in black beer produced 90 per cent fewer of these carcinogens than plain pork alone – with the dark brew showing a significantly greater protective effect than lighter-coloured lagers and non-alcoholic beers.

FEWER POLYPHENOLS   **MORE POLYPHENOLS**

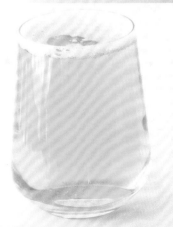
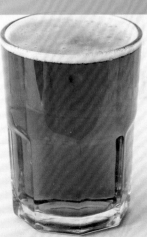
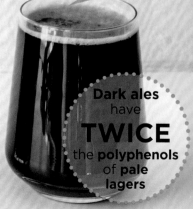

Dark ales have **TWICE** the **polyphenols** of **pale lagers**

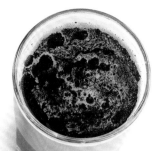

SIRLOIN STEAK IN SPICED BLACK BEER

Based on the formula used in the experiments at the University of Porto, but with my own special mix of sugars and spices, this simple marinade not only boosts the flavour and nutrients of the steak, but could also slash its levels of potential carcinogens too.

SERVES 2
PREP TIME 10 MINUTES, PLUS MARINATING
COOK TIME 5 MINUTES

....

2 SIRLOIN STEAKS

FOR THE MARINADE

200ML BLACK STOUT

2 TSP CLEAR HONEY

2 TSP SOY SAUCE

2 GARLIC CLOVES, MINCED

½ TSP MIXED SPICE

½ TSP DRIED OREGANO

½ TSP CHILLI FLAKES

½ TSP BLACK PEPPER

1 TBSP OLIVE OIL, PLUS EXTRA FOR FRYING

TO SERVE

TOASTED WHOLEGRAIN SOURDOUGH

SALAD LEAVES

FRIED RED ONIONS

MIXED SPICE

PAPRIKA

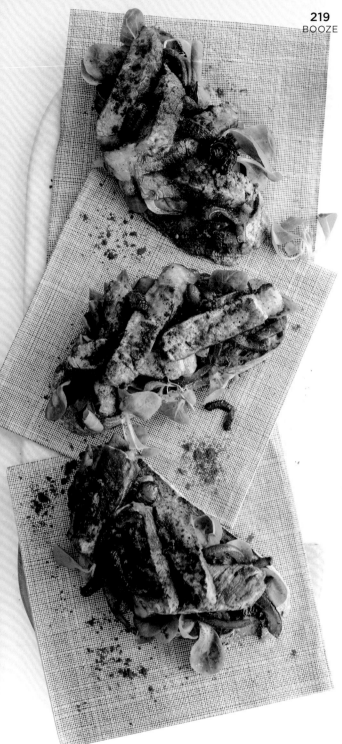

MIX all the marinade ingredients together in a plastic container. Add the steaks and toss to coat with the marinade. Cover and place in the fridge to marinate for at least 1 hour, but preferably overnight.

HEAT a little olive oil in a large frying pan until smoking. Remove the steaks from the marinade, allowing any excess liquid to drain off, and fry the steaks for 1½ minutes on each side for rare or 2½ minutes on each side for well done.

TRANSFER the steaks to a chopping board and let rest for 3 minutes before cutting into slices.

SERVE the slices of steak on toasted wholegrain sourdough with salad leaves and fried onions and a sprinkling of mixed spice and paprika.

INDEX

THE AUTHOR

James Wong is a Kew-trained botanist, science writer and broadcaster based in London. Graduating with a Master of Science degree in Ethnobotany in 2006, he pursued his key research interests of under-utilized crop species and traditional food systems through field work in rural Ecuador, Java and southern China.

He is the author of the best-selling books *Grow Your Drugs* and *Homegrown Revolution* as well as presenter of programmes including BBC2's award-winning *Grow Your Own Drugs* and the BBC's coverage of the world-renowned RHS Chelsea Flower Show. James is the co-presenter with Dr Michael Mosley of *The Secrets of Your Food*, a major BBC series on the science of food.

With his obsession for food almost eclipsing his love of plants, James's small London garden serves as a testing station for all manner of crops from around the world.

His first book for Mitchell Beazley, *RHS Grow for Flavour*, has sold 60,000 copies since first publication in spring 2015 and has been translated into 6 languages.

THE NUTRITIONAL CONSULTANT

Dr Emma Derbyshire, PhD, is a registered public health nutritionist and award-winning nutrition and health writer. She has a degree in Nutritional Biochemistry, a PhD in human nutrition and an experienced background in academia, research and advisory work.

Emma has written over 100 peer-reviewed publications, as well as contributing to scientific documents for the public sector, journal and healthcare articles and textbooks.

Emma is the founder of Nutritional Insight Limited, a consultancy to food and healthcare companies, Government organizations, top publishing houses, PR agencies and national newspapers.